A Comprehensive Guide with Healthy Recipes to Relieve IBS Symptoms

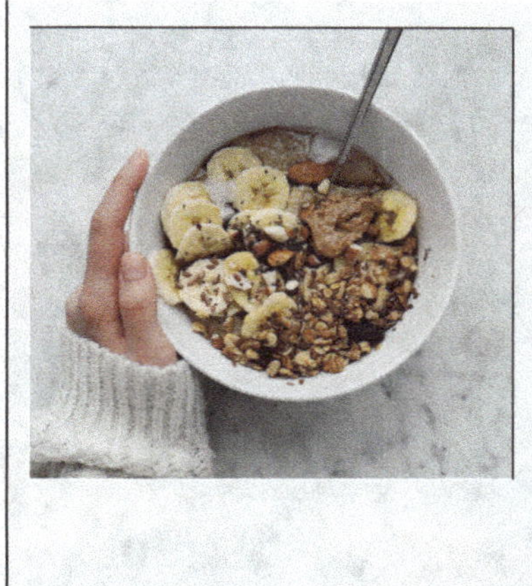

THE
LOW FODMAP
DIET

LINDA A. IVEY

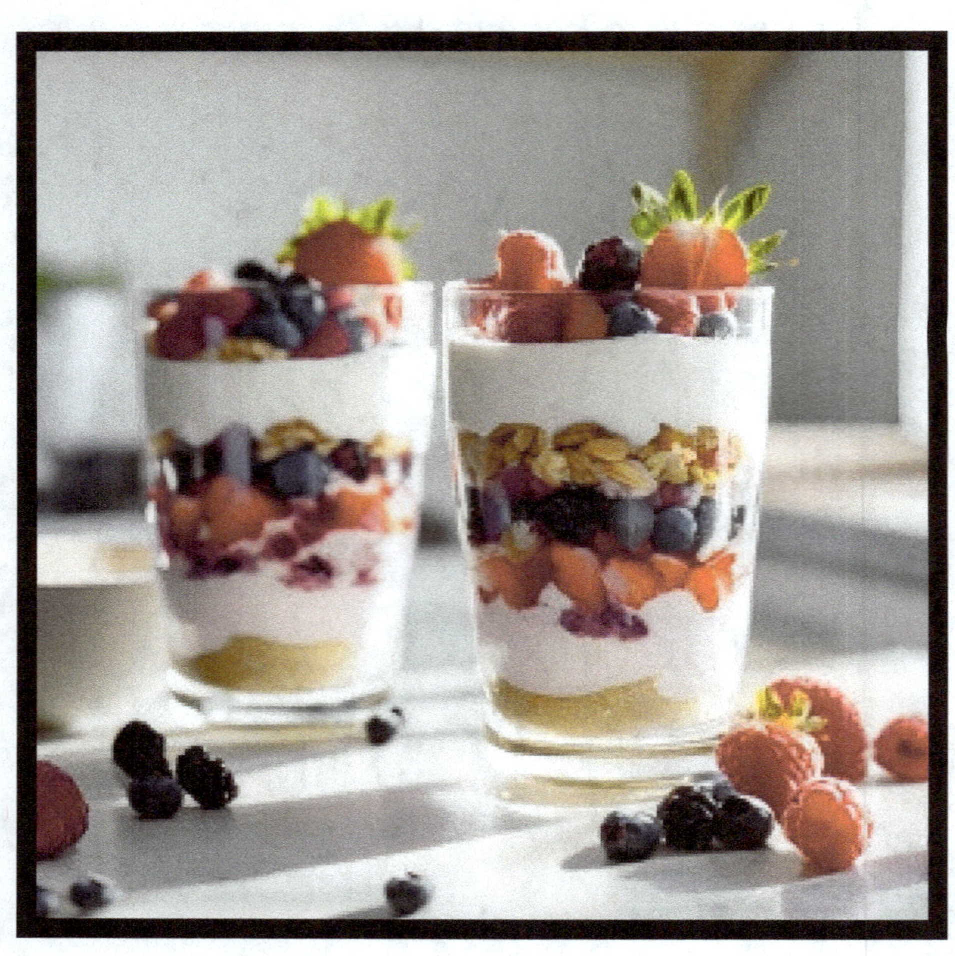

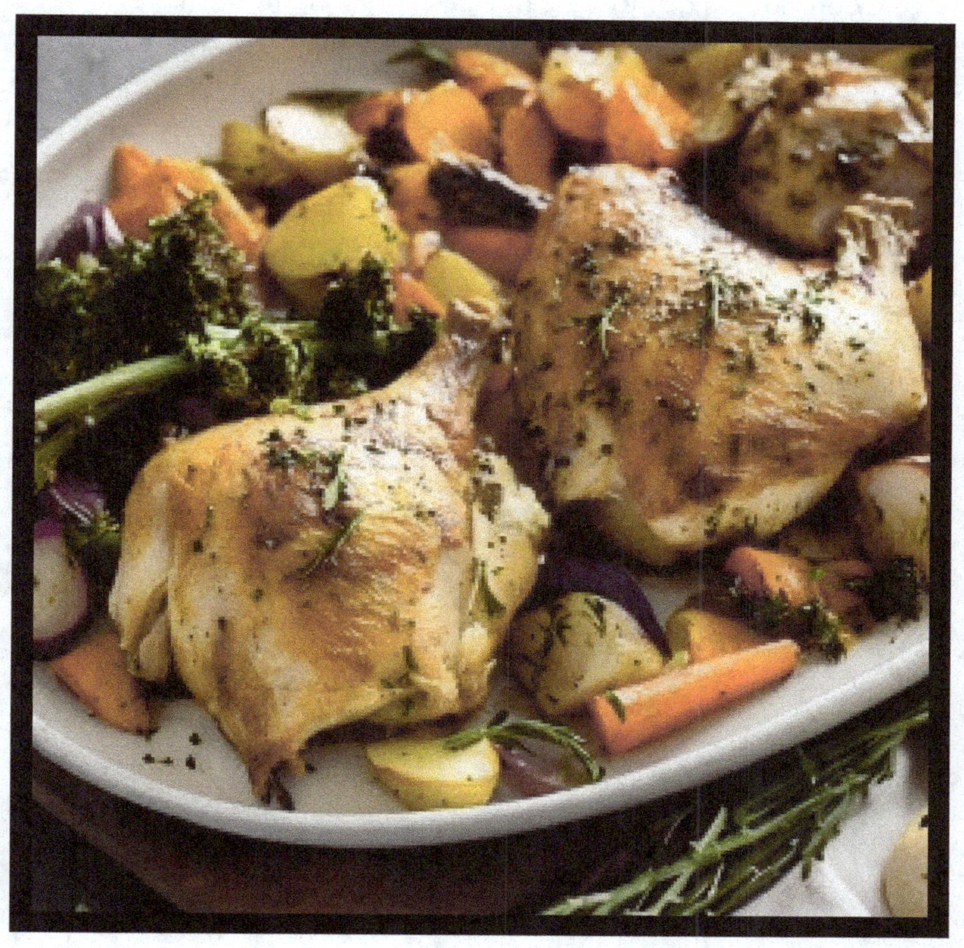

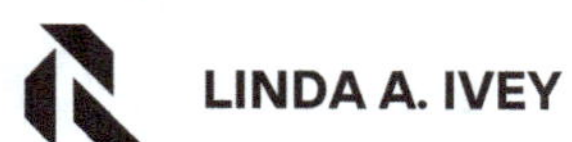

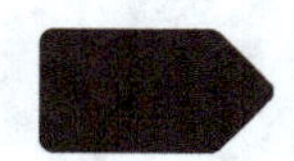

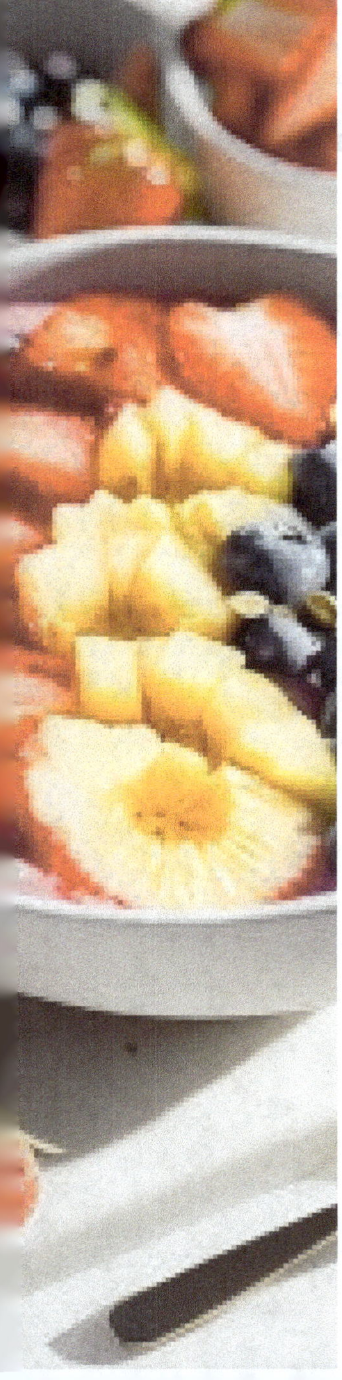

Table of Contents

Linda A. Ivey

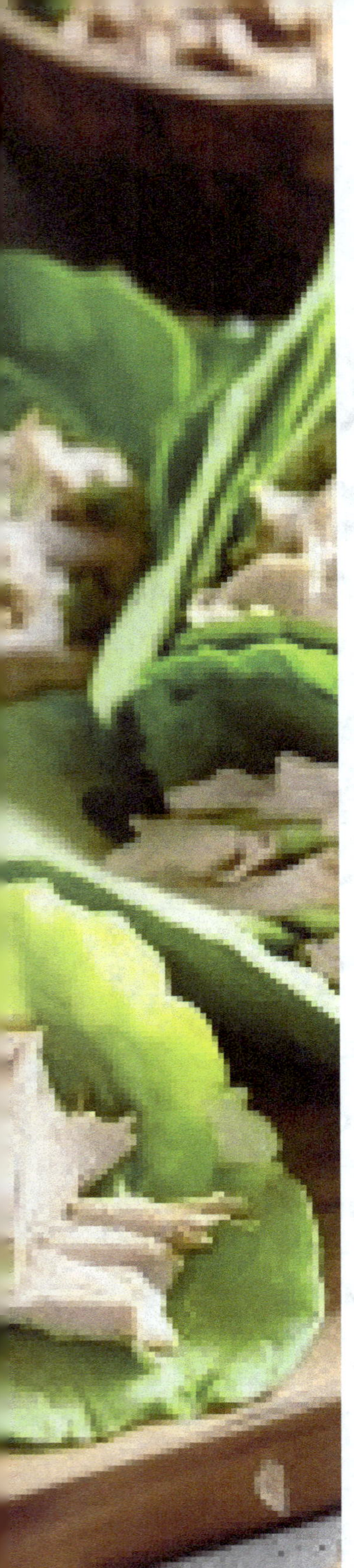

Linda A. Ivey

Introduction

Living with Irritable Bowel Syndrome (IBS) can feel like a daily battle, with unexpected bloating, abdominal pain, and digestive discomfort taking over your life. You're not alone—millions of people around the world face these daily challenges, trying to make sense of a gut that seems to rebel at every turn. The Low-FODMAP Diet has emerged as a scientifically proven way to help manage and even alleviate these troublesome symptoms, giving you a chance to take control of your gut health and enjoy food again.

This book, The Low-FODMAP Diet for Beginners, is your all-in-one guide to understanding and implementing this life-changing diet, designed especially for those who are new to the world of FODMAPs.

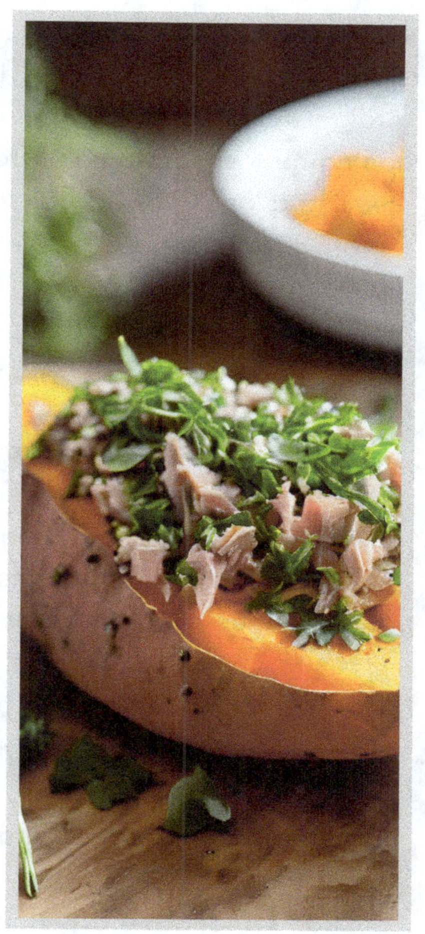

Our aim is simple: to empower you with the knowledge, tools, and recipes you need to soothe your digestive system and reclaim your daily comfort.

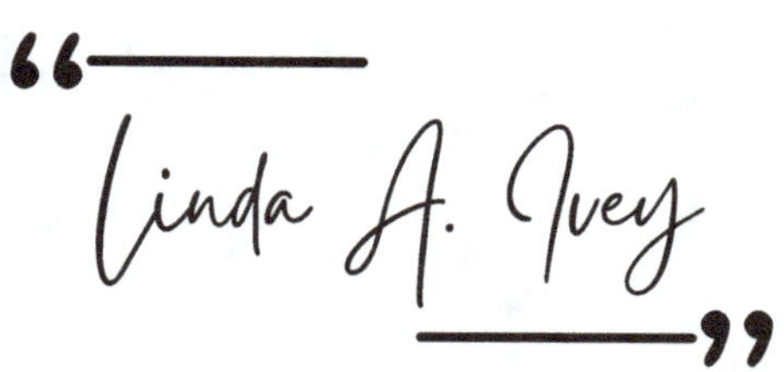

We understand that starting a new diet can be overwhelming, especially when it involves a complex network of foods that can either harm or heal your gut. That's why we've made every effort to simplify the Low-FODMAP Diet for you, breaking it down into digestible information and manageable steps. Whether you're hoping for immediate relief from distressing IBS symptoms or you're seeking a long-term strategy for maintaining gut health, this book provides a comprehensive approach tailored to your needs.

Inside, you'll discover:

1. What FODMAPs are and why they matter for people with IBS.
2. A step-by-step, 7-day meal plan with easy, delicious recipes to set you on the right path.
3. Practical advice for meal prep and grocery shopping, so you can make informed choices without the stress.
4. Guidance on reintroducing foods and customizing your diet to fit your lifestyle.
5. Tips for dining out and traveling, ensuring you can enjoy life without worrying about your next meal.

This book also recognizes that gut health isn't just about food—it's about how you feel, both physically and emotionally. We hope to provide not only dietary support but also a sense of reassurance, helping you find relief and gain confidence in your ability to manage IBS.

CHAPTER 1

WHAT FODMAPS ARE

If you suffer from Irritable Bowel Syndrome (IBS), you've likely noticed that certain foods seem to trigger symptoms like bloating, abdominal discomfort, and changes in bowel habits. But why do some foods affect you more than others? The answer often lies in FODMAPs—a term you may have heard but might not fully understand.

FODMAPs are a group of short-chain carbohydrates and sugar alcohols that are poorly absorbed in the small intestine. The acronym stands for Fermentable Oligosaccharides, Disaccharides, Monosaccharides, and Polyols. These specific types of carbohydrates are found in a wide range of foods, from certain fruits and vegetables to dairy products, grains, and sweeteners. While they may not cause issues for everyone, they can wreak havoc in the gut of someone with IBS or a sensitive digestive system.

To break it down further, here's what each component of FODMAPs entails:

1. **Oligosaccharides:** These include fructans (found in foods like wheat, garlic, and onions) and galacto-oligosaccharides (GOS) (present in legumes, lentils, and certain beans). Our bodies lack the enzymes to break these down, so they travel undigested to the large intestine, where they are fermented by gut bacteria, producing gas and causing bloating.

2. **Disaccharides:** The most common disaccharide linked to IBS symptoms is lactose, the sugar found in dairy products such as milk, cheese, and yogurt. People who are lactose intolerant don't produce enough lactase, the enzyme needed to break down lactose, which leads to digestive issues when they consume dairy.

3. **Monosaccharides:** Fructose is the monosaccharide of concern, and it's found in foods like honey, apples, mangoes, and high-fructose corn syrup. When there's an excess of fructose compared to glucose in the intestines, absorption can become problematic, causing symptoms like bloating and diarrhea.

4. **Polyols:** These are sugar alcohols, such as sorbitol, mannitol, xylitol, and maltitol, which occur naturally in some fruits and vegetables and are often used as artificial sweeteners. Polyols are poorly absorbed in the small intestine and can contribute to symptoms like bloating and stomach pain.

How FODMAPs Trigger Symptoms

For those with IBS or a sensitive gut, consuming high-FODMAP foods can be like lighting a match in a room full of gas. When these carbohydrates reach the large intestine without being properly digested, they become a feast for gut bacteria. As the bacteria ferment these carbohydrates, they produce gas, which can lead to bloating, discomfort, and distension of the abdomen. Furthermore, FODMAPs are highly osmotic, meaning they draw water into the intestines, which can lead to diarrhea in some cases or exacerbate constipation in others.

Why Understanding FODMAPs Is Important

Understanding FODMAPs is crucial for managing IBS symptoms effectively. By identifying which types of carbohydrates your gut struggles to digest, you can begin to make informed choices about your diet. It's important to note that not all FODMAPs will affect everyone in the same way. Your body might react strongly to one group of FODMAPs while tolerating another without issue. This is where the Low-FODMAP Diet comes in—helping you pinpoint your specific triggers and offering a personalized approach to relief.

By eliminating high-FODMAP foods from your diet for a short period and then gradually reintroducing them, you can discover which foods are causing your symptoms. Armed with this knowledge, you can tailor your diet to minimize discomfort and maximize your well-being.

HIGH AND LOW-FODMAP FOODS

What Makes a Food High or Low in FODMAPs?

The classification of foods into high or low FODMAPs depends on the concentration of specific short-chain carbohydrates present in them. High-FODMAP foods contain significant levels of fermentable carbohydrates, which, for those with IBS or a sensitive gut, can lead to symptoms such as bloating, pain, and irregular bowel movements. On the other hand, low-FODMAP foods contain minimal amounts of these carbohydrates and are generally easier to digest, making them less likely to trigger discomfort.

High-FODMAP Foods: Common Offenders

High-FODMAP foods are often rich in one or more of the fermentable carbohydrates that can irritate the gut. Here's a closer look at some common high-FODMAP foods across different categories:

- **Fruits:** Certain fruits are naturally high in fructose or polyols, which can be difficult for the gut to process. Examples include apples, pears, cherries, watermelon, mango, and stone fruits like peaches and plums.
- **Vegetables:** Vegetables like onions, garlic, cauliflower, asparagus, and artichokes are notorious for their high FODMAP content. These foods often contain fructans or mannitol, which can lead to digestive discomfort.

- **Legumes and Pulses:** Foods like chickpeas, lentils, kidney beans, and black beans are high in galacto-oligosaccharides (GOS), making them problematic for some individuals.
- **Grains:** Wheat, rye, and barley are common sources of fructans, found in foods such as bread, pasta, and cereals. These grains can be particularly challenging for those on a Low-FODMAP Diet.
- **Dairy:** Products like milk, soft cheeses, ice cream, and yogurt contain lactose, which can trigger symptoms for people who are lactose intolerant.
- **Sweeteners:** Artificial sweeteners like sorbitol, mannitol, xylitol, and maltitol, as well as natural sweeteners like honey and high-fructose corn syrup, are high in FODMAPs and may exacerbate gut issues.

Low-FODMAP Foods: Gut-Friendly Choices

In contrast, low-FODMAP foods are easier for the digestive system to handle, as they contain lower levels of fermentable carbohydrates. Incorporating these foods into your diet can help manage IBS symptoms and promote digestive comfort. Here are some examples:

- **Fruits:** While some fruits are high in FODMAPs, there are plenty of safe options. Bananas, strawberries, blueberries, oranges, grapes, and kiwis are low-FODMAP fruits that you can enjoy without triggering symptoms.
- **Vegetables:** Low-FODMAP vegetables include carrots, spinach, zucchini, potatoes, eggplant, bell peppers, and green beans. These options are gentle on the digestive tract and packed with nutrients.
- **Proteins:** Most animal-based proteins, such as chicken, beef, fish, eggs, and tofu (firm or silken), are naturally low in FODMAPs. They are excellent choices for meals that won't upset your gut.

Grains and Alternatives: Gluten-free grains like rice, quinoa, oats, and polenta are low in FODMAPs and provide a great base for many meals. Gluten-free bread and pasta options are also safe choices for those avoiding high-FODMAP grains.

- **Dairy Alternatives:** If you're lactose intolerant, you can enjoy dairy alternatives like lactose-free milk, almond milk, and hard cheeses like cheddar and Parmesan, which contain little to no lactose.
- **Nuts and Seeds:** Almonds, walnuts, chia seeds, and pumpkin seeds are nutritious, low-FODMAP options that add texture and healthy fats to your diet.

Why Differentiating Matters

Understanding which foods are high and low in FODMAPs is a crucial step in managing your diet effectively. It empowers you to make choices that minimize digestive discomfort and optimize your gut health. The goal of the Low-FODMAP Diet is not to restrict you permanently but to help you identify and eliminate the specific foods that trigger your symptoms, allowing you to reintroduce safe foods and enjoy a more balanced and enjoyable diet.

CHAPTER 2

THE LOW-FODMAP DIET EXPLAINED

Managing IBS symptoms can feel like navigating a complex maze, where every food choice seems to trigger discomfort. The Low-FODMAP Diet offers a structured, research-backed approach to alleviate symptoms and restore a sense of control over your digestive health. Central to this diet is a three-step process: Elimination, Reintroduction, and Maintenance. Let's dive into each phase and understand how they work together to help you identify your unique food triggers.

Step 1: Elimination

The Elimination phase is the first and most restrictive part of the Low-FODMAP Diet. During this step, you remove all high-FODMAP foods from your diet for a period of 4 to 8 weeks. This initial phase allows your gut to calm down and provides relief from IBS symptoms, as you eliminate the foods most likely to irritate your digestive system.

What to Avoid: High-FODMAP fruits, vegetables, grains, dairy, legumes, and sweeteners. This includes foods like apples, onions, wheat-based bread, cow's milk, and honey.

What to Eat: You'll focus on low-FODMAP alternatives, such as bananas, spinach, quinoa, lactose-free dairy, and lean proteins. The goal is to nourish your body with safe, digestible options.

The Purpose: This phase helps reduce symptoms, giving your digestive system a break and creating a clear baseline for comparison when you reintroduce foods later.

Note: It's important to work with a healthcare professional or dietitian during this phase to ensure you're meeting your nutritional needs while adhering to the diet's restrictions.

Step 2: Reintroduction

Once you experience symptom relief, you move into the Reintroduction phase. This step involves systematically reintroducing high-FODMAP foods back into your diet, one group at a time, to identify which specific carbohydrates trigger your symptoms.

How It Works: You'll reintroduce foods from each FODMAP group—oligosaccharides, disaccharides, monosaccharides, and polyols—one at a time. For example, you might start by testing foods high in fructans, like onions or garlic, while keeping the rest of your diet low in FODMAPs.

Monitoring Symptoms: After reintroducing each food, you'll carefully monitor your body's reaction. Note any bloating, pain, or other digestive issues, and track your symptoms in a food diary.

Adjusting Accordingly: If a food triggers symptoms, you'll know to limit or avoid it in the future. If a food doesn't cause any issues, it can be safely incorporated into your regular diet.

The Reintroduction phase is all about discovering your personal tolerance levels. Everyone's gut is unique, and this process empowers you to identify your specific triggers while expanding your food options as much as possible.

Step 3: Maintenance

The final phase, Maintenance, is where you create a personalized diet that supports your gut health and allows for a varied and enjoyable range of foods. By this point, you'll have a clearer understanding of which FODMAPs you can tolerate and which you should minimize or avoid.

Building Your Diet: Your diet will now be a balanced combination of low-FODMAP foods and the high-FODMAP foods you can tolerate without discomfort. This phase is about long-term sustainability and enjoying a diverse, nutritious diet while keeping your symptoms in check.

Living Flexibly: The Maintenance phase is not about strict restrictions but about finding a flexible and sustainable approach that works for your lifestyle. You'll have the confidence to make informed choices at home, when dining out, or while traveling, knowing how to manage your triggers.

Regular Check-Ins: As your digestive health may change over time, it's essential to reassess your diet periodically. New stressors, medications, or life changes might affect your symptoms, so being mindful and adaptive is key.

The Goal of the Three-Step Process

The purpose of the Low-FODMAP Diet is not to eliminate foods permanently but to empower you to make educated choices about what you eat. By following these three steps—Elimination, Reintroduction, and Maintenance—you can transform your approach to eating, reduce your IBS symptoms, and regain control over your quality of life. This method provides a structured path to better gut health while helping you understand your body's unique needs.

COMMON CHALLENGES

1. **Feeling Overwhelmed by Restrictions:** One of the biggest hurdles people face when starting the Low-FODMAP Diet is feeling overwhelmed by the sheer number of foods they need to avoid. Suddenly, familiar staples like bread, pasta, and even certain fruits and vegetables seem off-limits, making meal planning feel daunting.

2. **Dining Out and Social Situations:** Navigating restaurant menus and social gatherings can be tricky. The fear of unintentionally consuming a high-FODMAP ingredient often leads to anxiety, which can take the joy out of eating with friends or family.

3. **Missing Favorite Foods:** Giving up your favorite high-FODMAP foods, even temporarily, can be emotionally challenging. The cravings for familiar comfort foods may make sticking to the diet feel even harder.

4. **Grocery Shopping Confusion:** Reading food labels and understanding which ingredients to avoid can be confusing. Many packaged foods contain hidden FODMAPs, making the shopping experience stressful and time-consuming.

5. **Staying Motivated and Consistent:** The diet's restrictive nature can feel like a test of willpower, especially if you don't experience immediate symptom relief. It's easy to feel discouraged and tempted to give up.

STRATEGIES FOR A SMOOTH START

Overcoming these challenges requires preparation, patience, and a bit of creativity. Here are some practical strategies to help you get off to a successful start:

1. **Educate Yourself Thoroughly:** Take the time to learn about FODMAPs and which foods are high and low in them. Understanding the science behind the diet can help you feel more in control and less anxious about the restrictions. Keep a printed or digital list of low-FODMAP foods handy as a quick reference.

2. **Plan Your Meals and Snacks:** Meal planning is a game-changer for staying organized and reducing stress. At the start of each week, map out your meals and snacks, make a detailed grocery list, and prep ingredients in advance. Having ready-to-go, low-FODMAP meals will help you avoid last-minute, high-FODMAP temptations.

3. **Stock Your Pantry with Essentials:** Fill your kitchen with versatile low-FODMAP staples, such as gluten-free grains (like rice and quinoa), canned tuna, lactose-free dairy, and fresh, low-FODMAP fruits and vegetables. This way, you'll always have ingredients on hand for a quick, satisfying meal.

4. **Simplify Your Recipes:** When you're first starting out, stick to simple recipes with minimal ingredients. Basic, easy-to-prepare meals, like grilled chicken with roasted carrots and potatoes, can be just as delicious as more elaborate dishes. As you gain confidence, you can experiment with more complex low-FODMAP recipes.

5. **Be Strategic When Eating Out:** Before dining at a restaurant, research the menu and call ahead to ask about ingredient options. Many restaurants are willing to accommodate dietary needs if you make a request in advance. Choose dishes that are naturally low in FODMAPs, such as grilled meats and plain vegetables, and ask for dressings or sauces on the side.

6. **Communicate with Friends and Family:** Let your loved ones know about your dietary restrictions and why you're following the Low-FODMAP Diet. A supportive environment can make social situations less stressful. Offer to bring a dish you know you can eat to gatherings so that you have at least one safe option.

7. **Find Low-FODMAP Alternatives for Favorite Foods:** Missing your favorite high-FODMAP foods can be tough, but there are plenty of delicious substitutes. For example, you can use gluten-free bread instead of wheat bread or lactose-free yogurt in place of regular yogurt. Experiment with low-FODMAP seasonings and flavors to make your meals enjoyable.

8. **Track Your Progress and Symptoms:** Keeping a food and symptom diary can help you stay on track and make the connection between what you eat and how you feel. Recording your progress can also be motivating, especially when you start noticing improvements in your symptoms.

9. **Stay Patient and Flexible:** Remember that the Low-FODMAP Diet is a journey, not a quick fix. It may take time for your symptoms to improve and for you to get used to the changes. Be patient with yourself and flexible in your approach—if something isn't working, don't be afraid to adjust your strategy.

10. **Seek Professional Support:** Working with a registered dietitian who specializes in the Low-FODMAP Diet can make a world of difference. They can provide personalized guidance, help you stay nutritionally balanced, and troubleshoot any challenges you encounter.

Starting the Low-FODMAP Diet can be challenging, but it's also an opportunity to gain a deeper understanding of your body and take control of your gut health.

By approaching the diet with preparation, flexibility, and a positive attitude, you'll be better equipped to handle obstacles and experience the relief you're hoping for. Remember, every small step you take is progress, and the journey is about finding what works best for you.

PREPARING FOR SUCCESS

When embarking on the Low-FODMAP Diet, preparation is key to making your journey smooth and effective. The diet may seem overwhelming at first, but with the right strategies in place, you'll feel more confident and motivated to follow through. Preparing for success means equipping yourself with the knowledge, tools, and mindset needed to navigate your new way of eating. Let's explore how to set yourself up for long-term success.

Tips for Planning Your Meals

Meal planning is one of the most powerful tools you can use to simplify the Low-FODMAP Diet and reduce stress around food choices. Taking the time to plan your meals ensures that you're always prepared and have plenty of safe, nutritious options available. Here's how to make meal planning work for you:

1. **Start with a Weekly Meal Plan:** Dedicate time each week to map out your breakfasts, lunches, dinners, and snacks. This will help you stay organized, avoid last-minute decisions, and reduce the temptation to reach for high-FODMAP foods.

2. **Focus on Variety:** Eating the same meals repeatedly can get boring, so aim to include a mix of proteins, vegetables, grains, and healthy fats in your meal plan. This will keep your meals exciting and help you get a balanced array of nutrients.

3. **Batch Cooking and Meal Prep:** Cook larger portions of your favorite meals and store them in the refrigerator or freezer. This way, you'll always have something ready to eat, even on busy days. Soups, casseroles, and roasted vegetables are great for batch cooking.

4. **Use Leftovers Wisely:** Repurpose leftovers into new meals. For example, grilled chicken from dinner can become a tasty salad topping for lunch the next day.

5. **Keep Your Meals Balanced:** Each meal should contain a protein source, a low-FODMAP vegetable, and a serving of healthy carbohydrates. This balance will keep you satisfied and energized throughout the day.

GROCERY SHOPPING MADE SIMPLE

Navigating the grocery store while following the Low-FODMAP Diet can be tricky, but a bit of preparation will make the experience much smoother. Here are some strategies for efficient and stress-free grocery shopping:

1. **Make a Detailed Shopping List:** Write down all the ingredients you need for the week based on your meal plan. Organize your list by category (e.g., produce, proteins, pantry staples) to make your shopping trip more efficient.

2. **Focus on Whole, Unprocessed Foods:** Fresh vegetables, fruits, lean proteins, and gluten-free grains are often the safest options. Avoid packaged and processed foods, as they may contain hidden FODMAPs.

3. **Read Labels Carefully:** Check ingredient lists for high-FODMAP additives like high-fructose corn syrup, garlic, onion powder, or inulin. Familiarize yourself with the names of common FODMAPs so you can easily identify them.

4. **Stock Up on Low-FODMAP Staples:** Keep your pantry stocked with essentials like rice, quinoa, gluten-free pasta, canned tuna, lactose-free dairy, and low-FODMAP snacks. Having these staples on hand will make meal prep faster and more convenient.

5. **Shop Seasonally:** Choose fruits and vegetables that are in season for the best flavor and affordability. This will also help you incorporate more variety into your meals.

To make meal prep as efficient and enjoyable as possible, having the right kitchen tools and equipment is essential. Here are some must-haves to set you up for meal prep success:

1. **Quality Knives and a Cutting Board:** A sharp knife and a sturdy cutting board make chopping vegetables and proteins much easier. Invest in a chef's knife and a smaller paring knife for more precise tasks.

2. **Food Storage Containers:** Use a variety of containers in different sizes to store prepped ingredients and leftovers. Glass containers are great for reheating meals and are environmentally friendly.

3. **A Slow Cooker or Instant Pot:** These appliances can save you time and effort by making one-pot meals with minimal prep. Perfect for soups, stews, and large batches of grains.

4. **A Spiralizer:** For those who enjoy vegetable-based dishes, a spiralizer can turn zucchinis, carrots, and other veggies into noodles for a fun and healthy pasta alternative.

5. **Measuring Cups and Spoons:** Precision is crucial in baking and cooking, especially when following recipes that need to stay Low-FODMAP. Keep measuring tools on hand to ensure accuracy.

6. **Baking Sheets and Parchment Paper:** Roasting vegetables and proteins is a simple and tasty way to prepare meals. Parchment paper makes cleanup a breeze.

7. **Blender or Food Processor:** Great for making smoothies, hummus, sauces, and soups. It's a versatile tool that can help you create a variety of delicious Low-FODMAP dishes.

Putting It All Together

Preparing for success on the Low-FODMAP Diet is about making your life easier, not harder. By planning your meals, simplifying your grocery shopping routine, and investing in essential kitchen tools, you'll feel more in control and better equipped to manage your diet.

The more organized and prepared you are, the less stressful and more enjoyable your journey will be.

Remember, small steps add up to big changes. Take it one day at a time, and don't be afraid to experiment with new ingredients and flavors. With these strategies, you're well on your way to achieving your gut health goals.

CHAPTER 4

BREAKFAST RECIPES

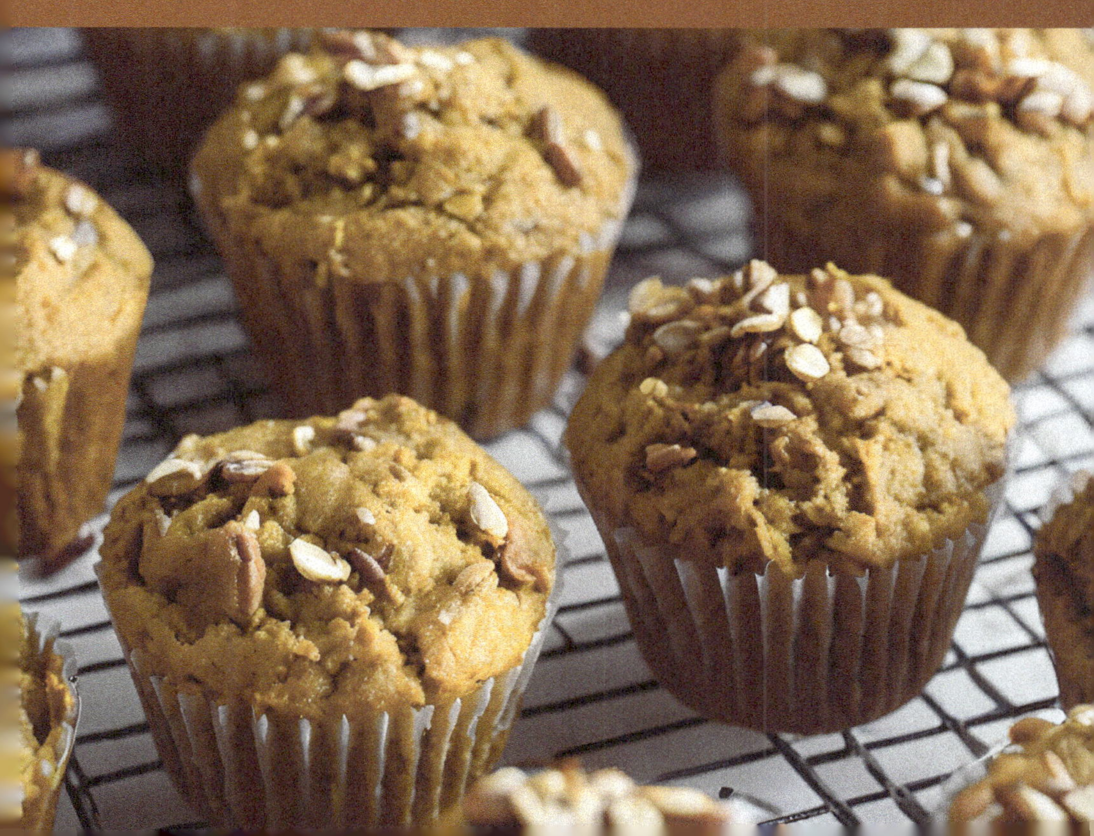

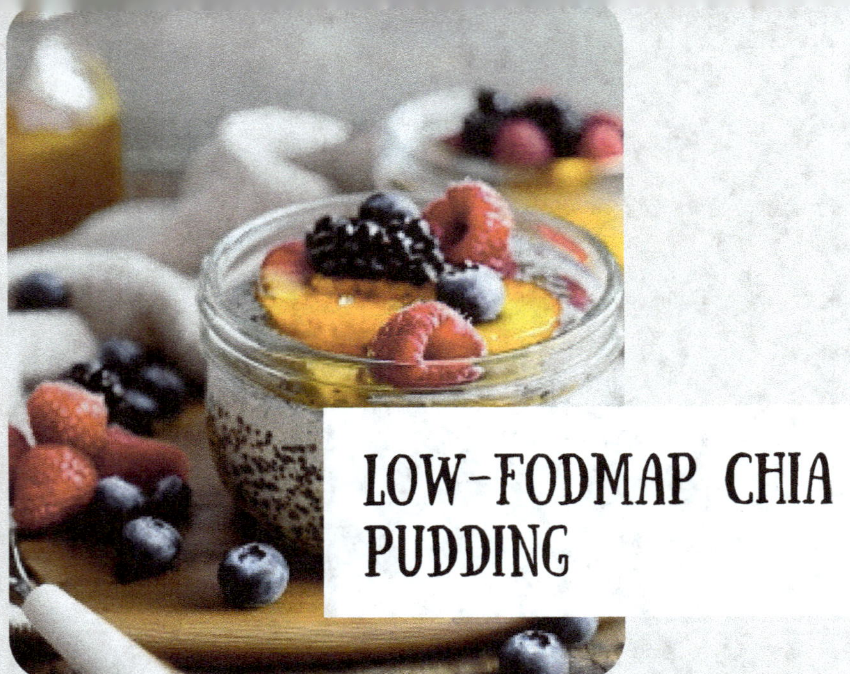

LOW-FODMAP CHIA PUDDING

SERVINGS: 2   PREPPING TIME: 5 MINUTES (PLUS 2 HOURS OR OVERNIGHT CHILLING)

INGREDIENTS

1/4 cup chia seeds

1 cup lactose-free milk or almond milk

1 tablespoon maple syrup

Fresh strawberries or blueberries for topping

DIRECTIONS

1. In a bowl or jar, mix chia seeds, lactose-free milk, and maple syrup. Stir well.
2. Cover and refrigerate for at least 2 hours or overnight, stirring occasionally.
3. Serve chilled with fresh berries on top.

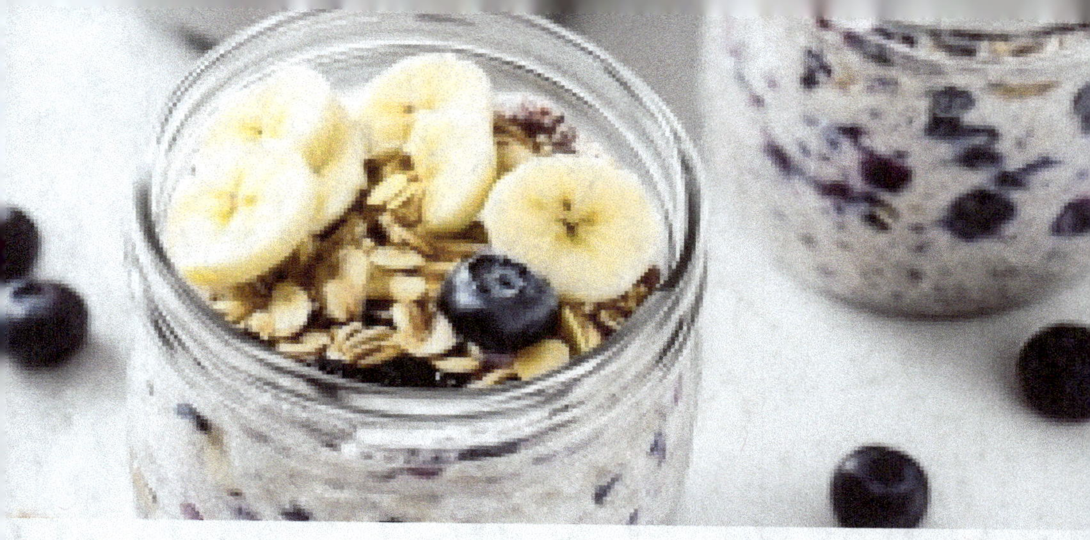

Banana and Blueberry Overnight Oats

Ingredients :

1 cup gluten-free rolled oats

1 1/2 cups lactose-free milk or
almond milk

1 medium ripe banana, sliced

1/2 cup fresh blueberries

1 tablespoon chia seeds

1 teaspoon maple syrup (optional)

A pinch of cinnamon (optional)

Procedure :

1. In a large bowl or mason jar,
combine oats, lactose-free milk,
sliced banana, blueberries, and chia
seeds. Stir well.

2. Add maple syrup and cinnamon if
desired.

3. Cover and refrigerate overnight.

4. In the morning, give the mixture
a good stir and enjoy cold or
warmed up.

Prep Time : 5 minutes
plus overnight soaking

Servings : 2

Savory Breakfast Quinoa Bowl

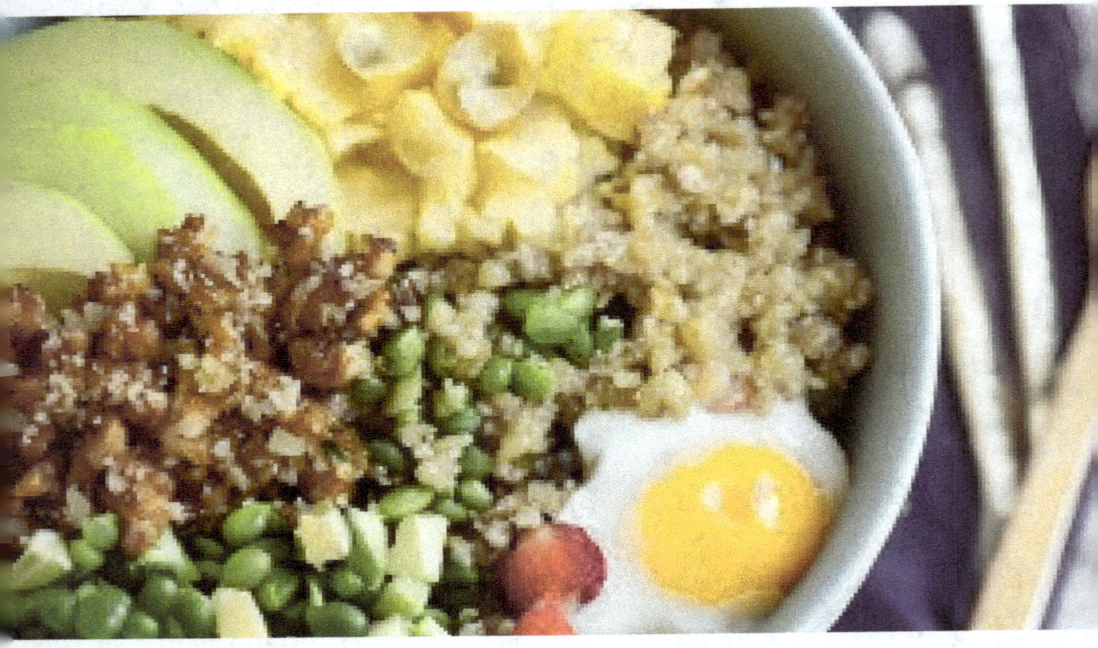

 2 servings    15 minutes

INGREDIENTS

1 cup cooked quinoa

2 large eggs, fried or poached

1/2 avocado, sliced

1/4 cup diced tomatoes

Salt and pepper to taste

DIRECTIONS

1. Divide cooked quinoa between two bowls.
2. Top each bowl with a fried or poached egg, avocado slices, and diced tomatoes.
3. Season with salt and pepper.

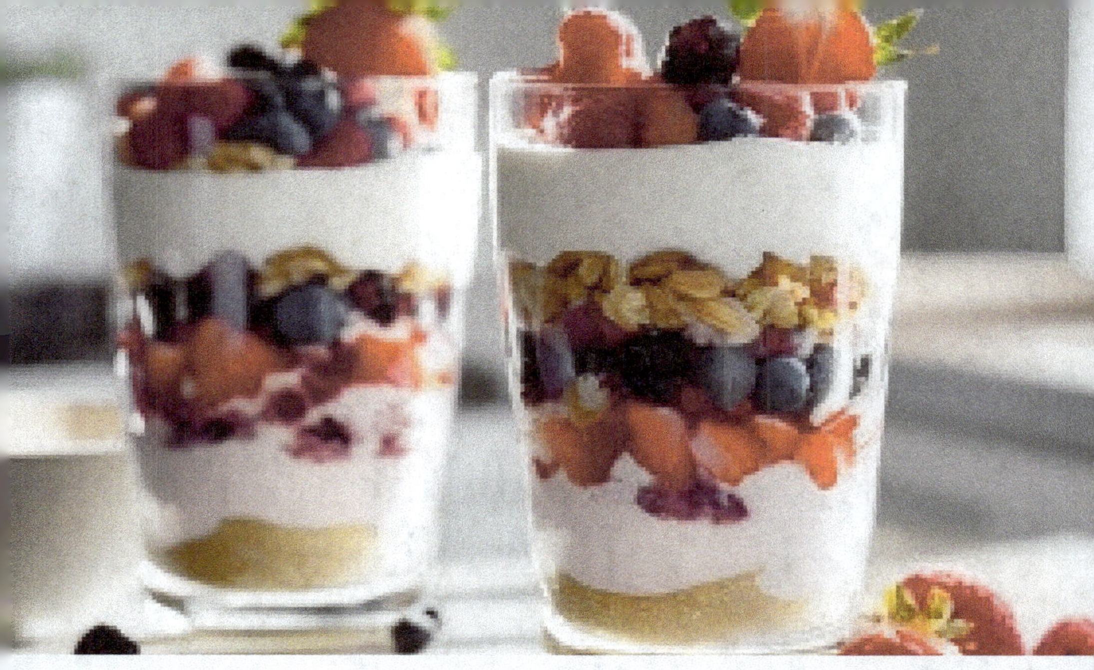

Low-FODMAP Berry Parfait

Ingredients :

1 cup lactose-free yogurt

1/2 cup strawberries, sliced

1/2 cup blueberries

1/4 cup gluten-free granola

Procedure :

1. In a glass or bowl, layer lactose-free yogurt, sliced strawberries, blueberries, and gluten-free granola.

2. Repeat layers and serve immediately.

Prep Time : 5 minutes

Servings : 2

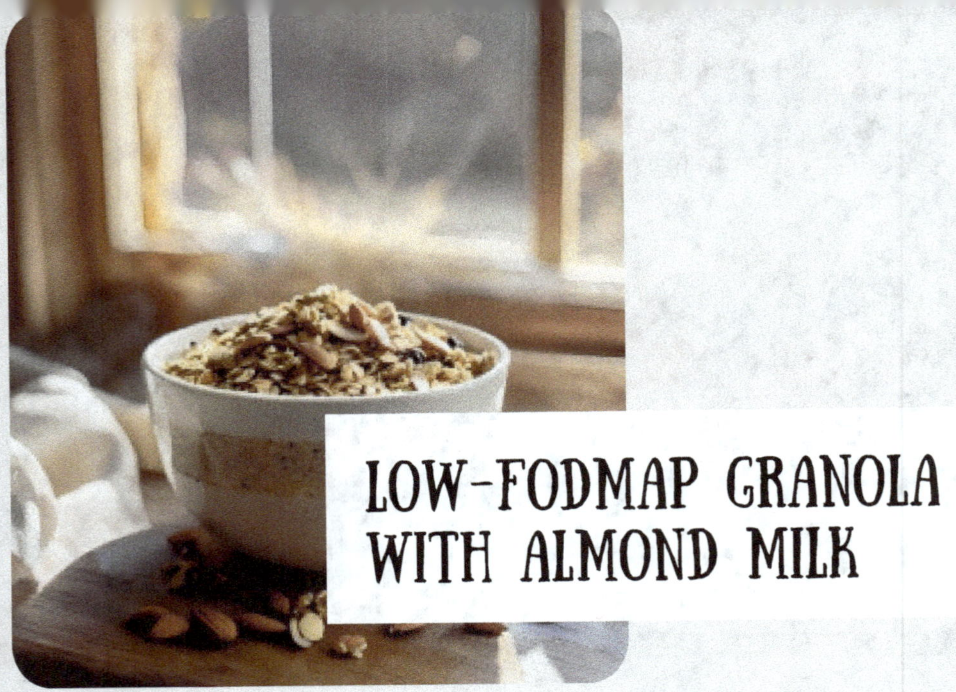

LOW-FODMAP GRANOLA WITH ALMOND MILK

SERVINGS: 4

COOKING TIME: 30 MIN

INGREDIENTS

2 cups gluten-free rolled oats

1/2 cup chopped walnuts

1/4 cup shredded coconut

1/4 cup maple syrup

2 tablespoons olive oil

1 teaspoon vanilla extract

DIRECTIONS

1. Preheat oven to 300°F (150°C).
2. In a bowl, mix oats, walnuts, shredded coconut, maple syrup, olive oil, and vanilla extract.
3. Spread the mixture on a baking sheet and bake for 25-30 minutes, stirring halfway through.
4. Let cool and serve with almond milk.

Pumpkin Spice Breakfast Muffins

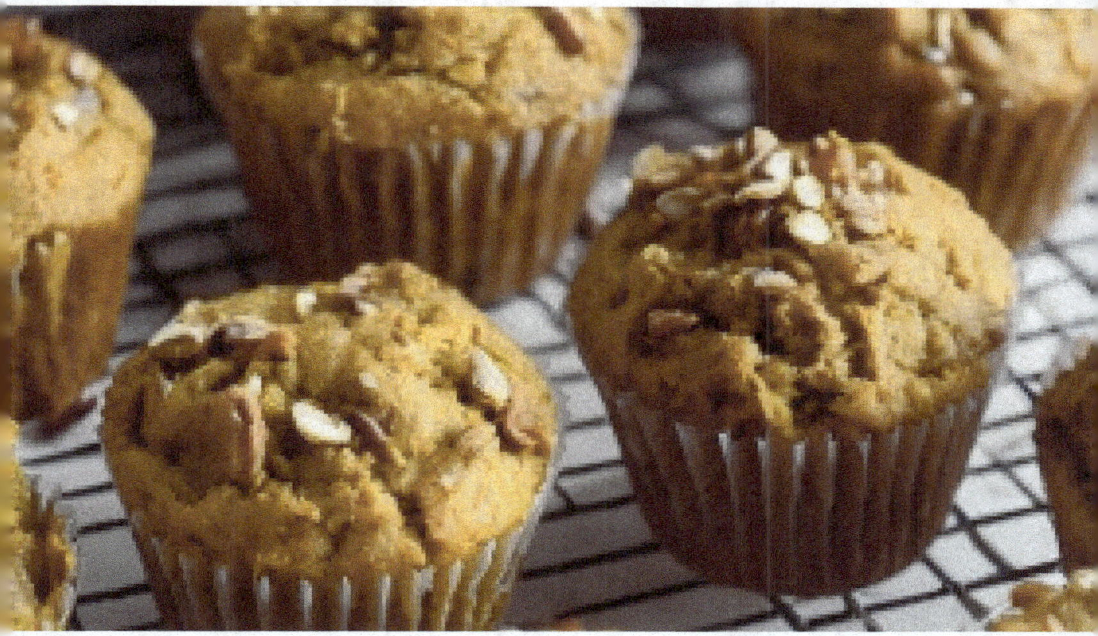

 12 muffins   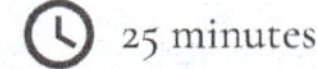 25 minutes

INGREDIENTS

2 cups gluten-free flour

1 cup canned pumpkin
puree

1/2 cup lactose-free
milk

1/2 cup maple syrup

2 large eggs

1 teaspoon baking
powder

1 teaspoon cinnamon

DIRECTIONS

1. Preheat oven to 350°F (175°C) and line a muffin tin with paper liners.
2. In a bowl, combine all ingredients and mix until smooth.
3. Divide the batter evenly among the muffin cups and bake for 20–25 minutes, or until a toothpick comes out clean.

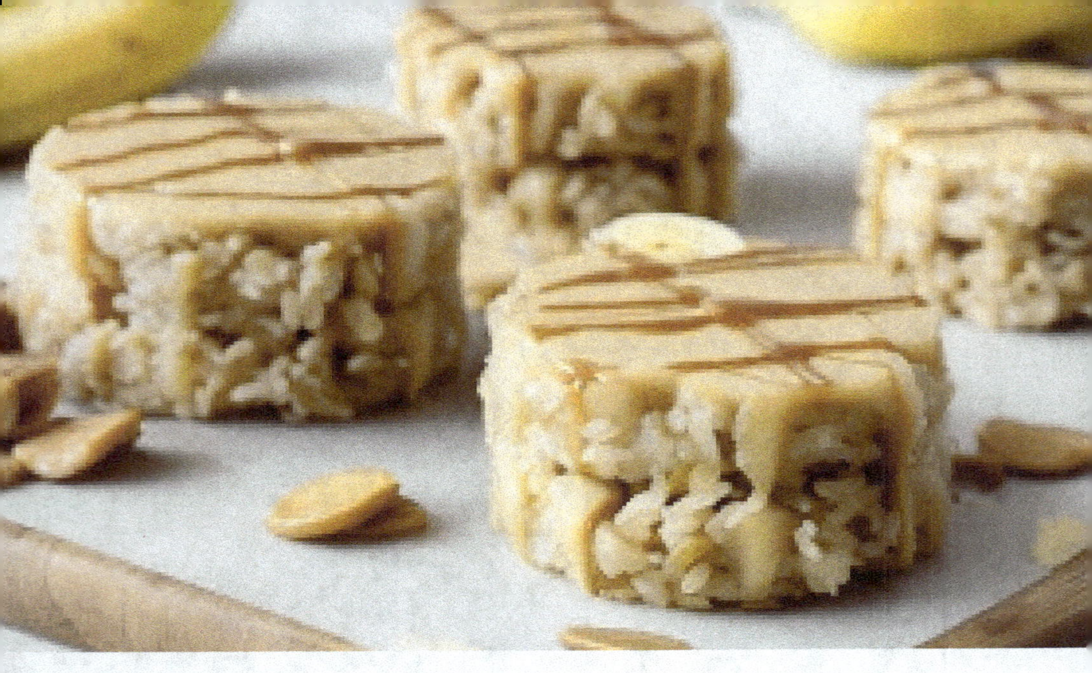

Peanut Butter Banana Rice Cakes

Ingredients :

2 rice cakes

2 tablespoons peanut butter

1 medium banana, sliced

A sprinkle of cinnamon

Procedure :

1. Spread peanut butter evenly over each rice cake.

2. Top with banana slices and a sprinkle of cinnamon.

Prep Time : 5 minutes

Servings : 2

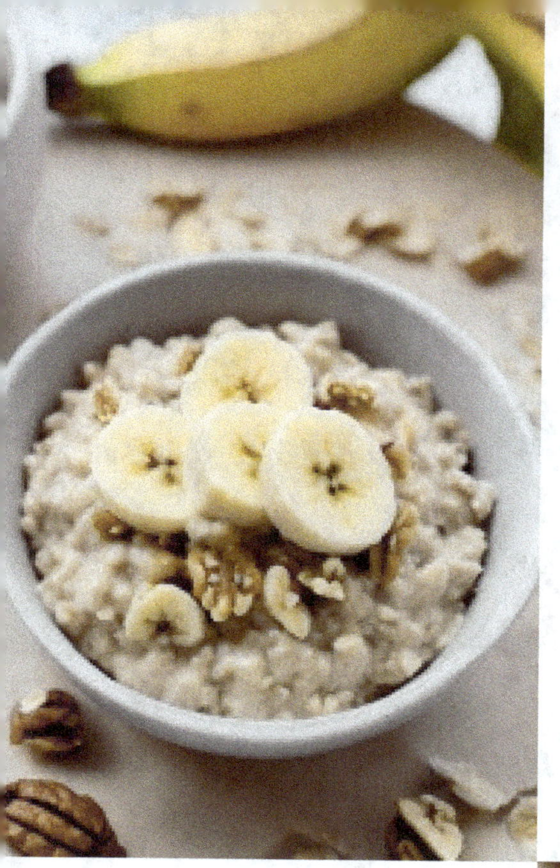

Oatmeal with Banana and Walnuts

 1 servings    10 minutes

INGREDIENTS

1/2 cup gluten-free rolled oats

1 cup lactose-free milk or water

1 banana, sliced

2 tablespoons chopped walnuts

1 tablespoon maple syrup

(optional)

DIRECTIONS

1. Cook oats in lactose-free milk or water according to package instructions.

2. Top with banana slices, chopped walnuts, and maple syrup if desired.

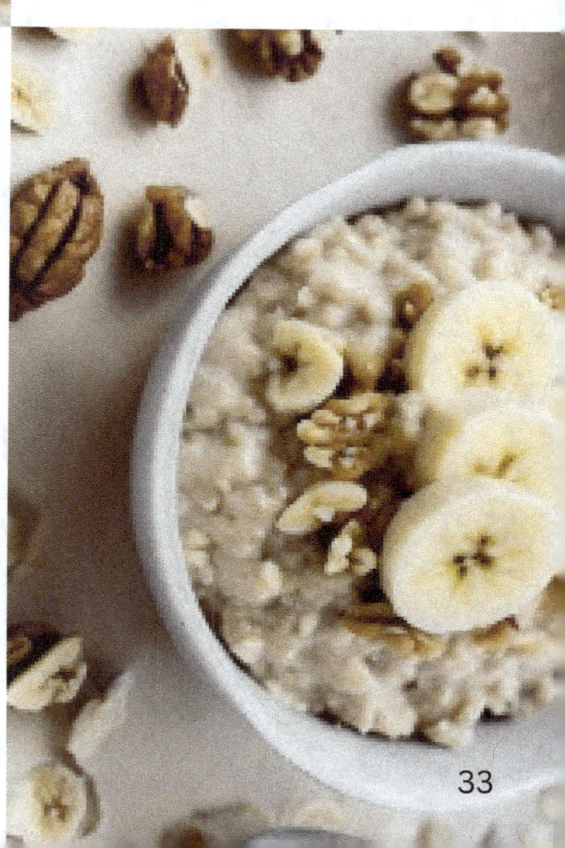

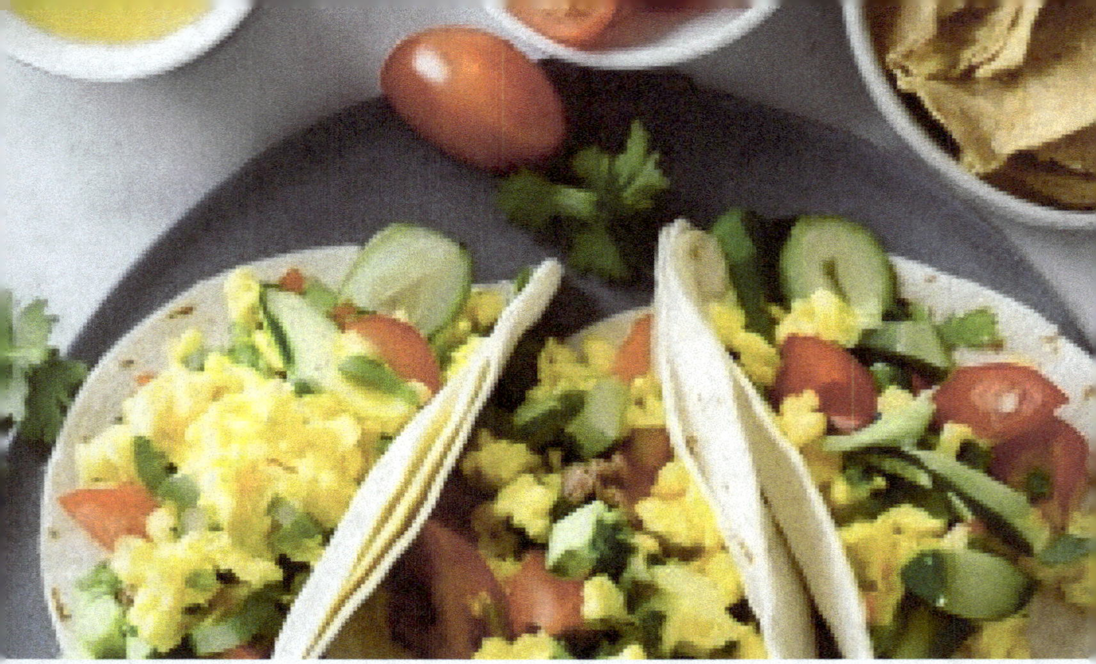

Breakfast Tacos with Scrambled Eggs and Vegetables

Ingredients :

4 corn tortillas

4 large eggs

1/2 cup diced bell peppers

1/2 cup diced zucchini

1 tablespoon olive oil

Salt and pepper to taste

Prep Time : 15 minutes

Servings : 2

Procedure :

1. Heat olive oil in a pan over medium heat. Add diced bell peppers and zucchini, cooking until tender.

2. In a bowl, whisk eggs with salt and pepper, then add to the pan. Cook until scrambled and set.

3. Warm the corn tortillas and fill each with scrambled eggs and vegetables.

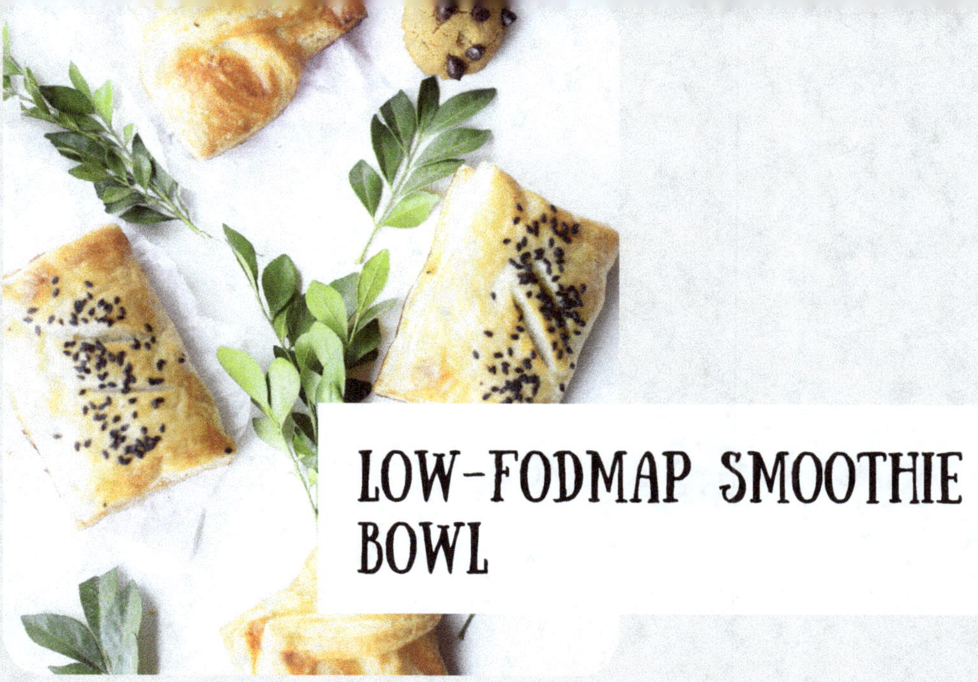

LOW-FODMAP SMOOTHIE BOWL

SERVINGS: 1   PREPPING TIME: 5 MIN   COOKING TIME: 0 MIN

INGREDIENTS

1 frozen banana

1/2 cup frozen strawberries

1/2 cup lactose-free yogurt

1 tablespoon peanut butter (without added sugar)

1/4 cup almond milk

Toppings: sliced kiwi, coconut flakes, chia seeds

DIRECTIONS

1. In a blender, combine the frozen banana, strawberries, lactose-free yogurt, peanut butter, and almond milk. Blend until smooth.
2. Pour into a bowl and top with kiwi slices, coconut flakes, and chia seeds.

CHAPTER 5

LUNCH RECIPES

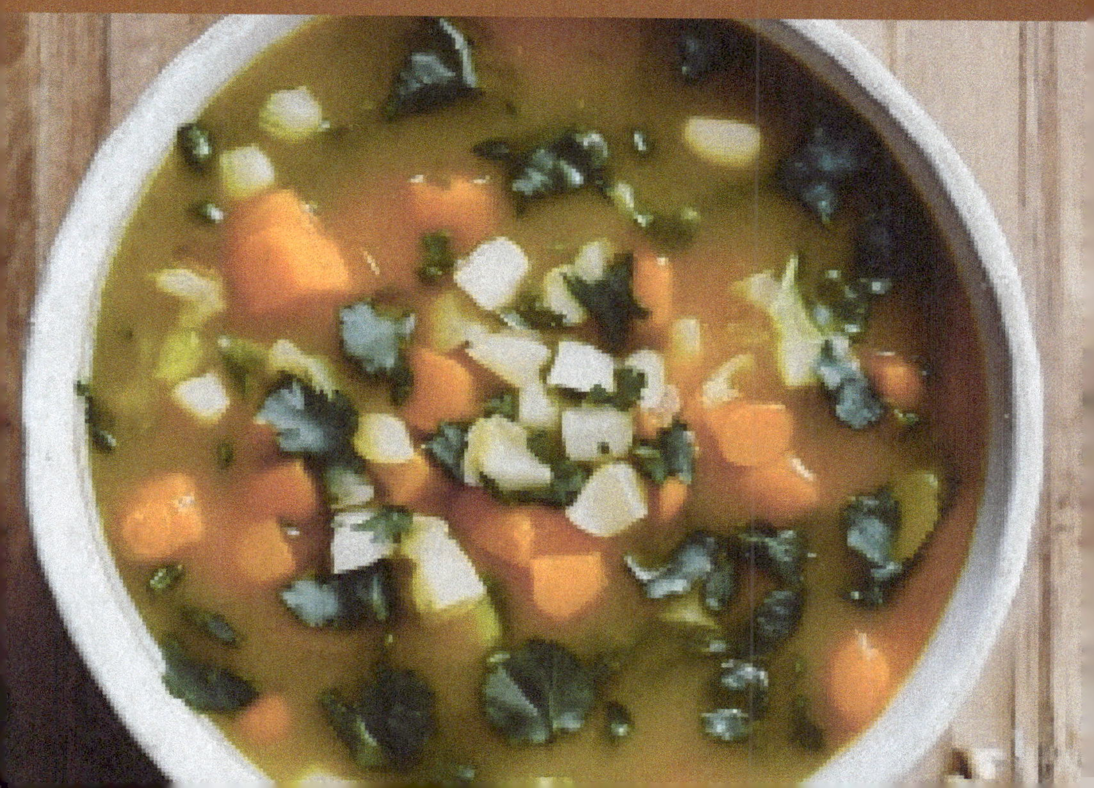

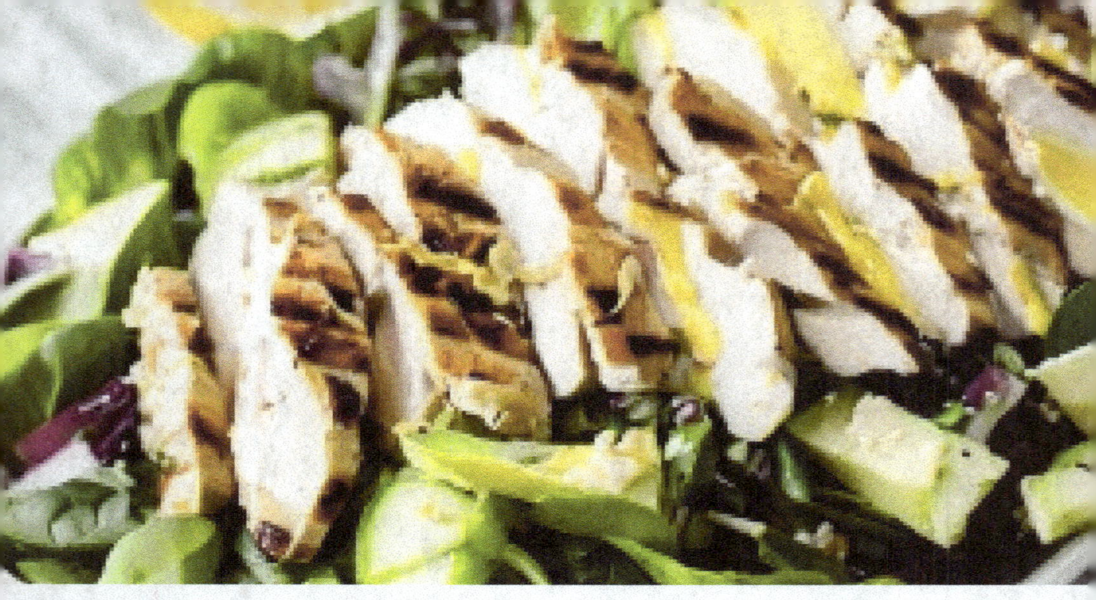

Grilled Chicken Salad with Lemon Vinaigrette

Ingredients :

2 boneless, skinless chicken
breasts
4 cups mixed salad greens
1/2 cucumber, sliced
1/2 cup cherry tomatoes, halved
1/4 cup crumbled feta cheese
(optional)
2 tablespoons olive oil
Juice of 1 lemon
Salt and pepper to taste

Prep Time : 20 minutes

Servings : 2

Procedure :

1. Season chicken breasts with salt
and pepper. Grill or pan-sear over
medium heat until fully cooked,
about 6-8 minutes per side.

2. In a large bowl, combine salad
greens, cucumber, cherry
tomatoes, and feta cheese.

3. Slice the cooked chicken and
add to the salad.

4. In a small bowl, whisk olive oil
and lemon juice. Drizzle over the
salad and toss to coat.

Lactose-Free Caprese Salad

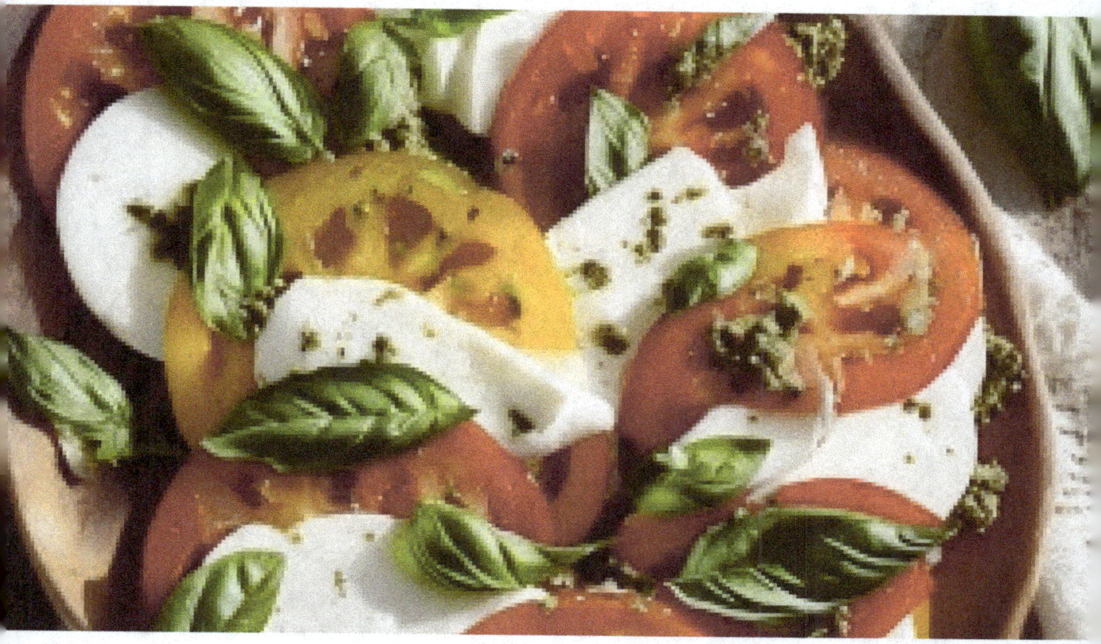

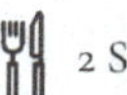 2 Servings 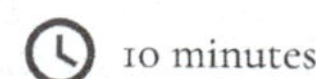 10 minutes

INGREDIENTS

2 large tomatoes, sliced
8 ounces lactose-free
mozzarella, sliced
Fresh basil leaves
2 tablespoons olive oil
Balsamic vinegar to taste
Salt and pepper to taste

DIRECTIONS

1. Layer tomato slices, mozzarella slices, and basil leaves on a plate.
2. Drizzle with olive oil and balsamic vinegar. Season with salt and pepper.

Asian-Inspired Rice Noodle Salad

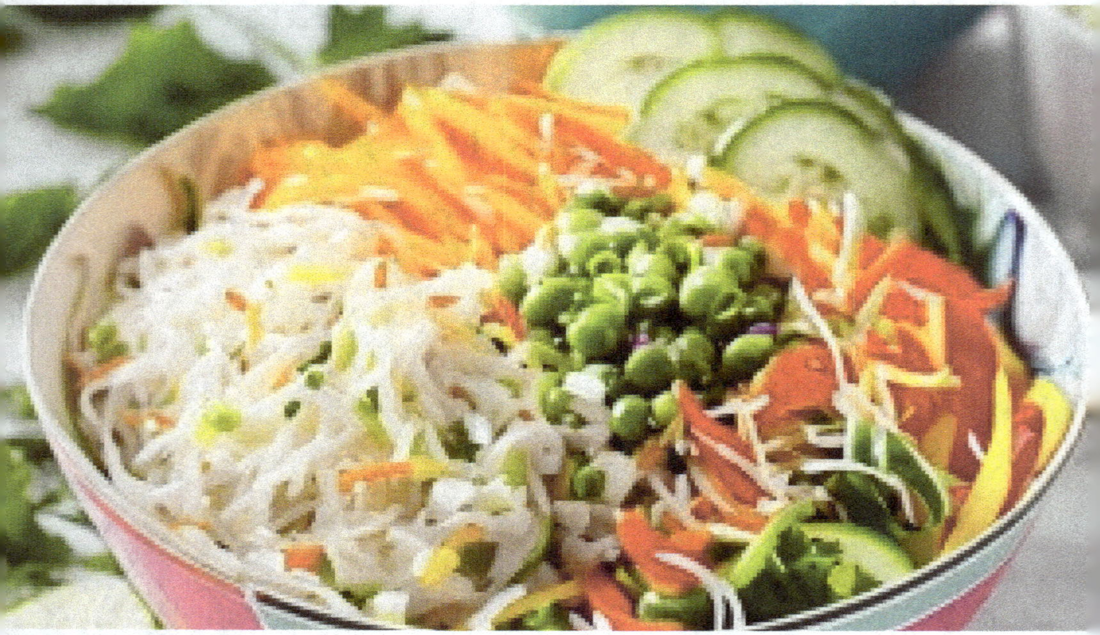

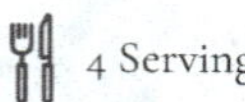 4 Servings 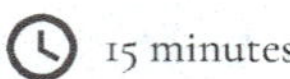 15 minutes

INGREDIENTS

8 ounces rice noodles
1/2 cup shredded carrots
1/2 cup sliced bell peppers
1/4 cup chopped scallions
(green parts only)
1 tablespoon sesame oil
2 tablespoons tamari
(gluten-free soy sauce)
Juice of 1 lime

DIRECTIONS

1. Cook rice noodles according to package instructions. Drain and rinse with cold water.

2. In a large bowl, combine noodles, carrots, bell peppers, and scallions.

3. In a small bowl, mix sesame oil, tamari, and lime juice. Pour over the salad and toss to coat.

Turkey and Avocado Lettuce Wraps

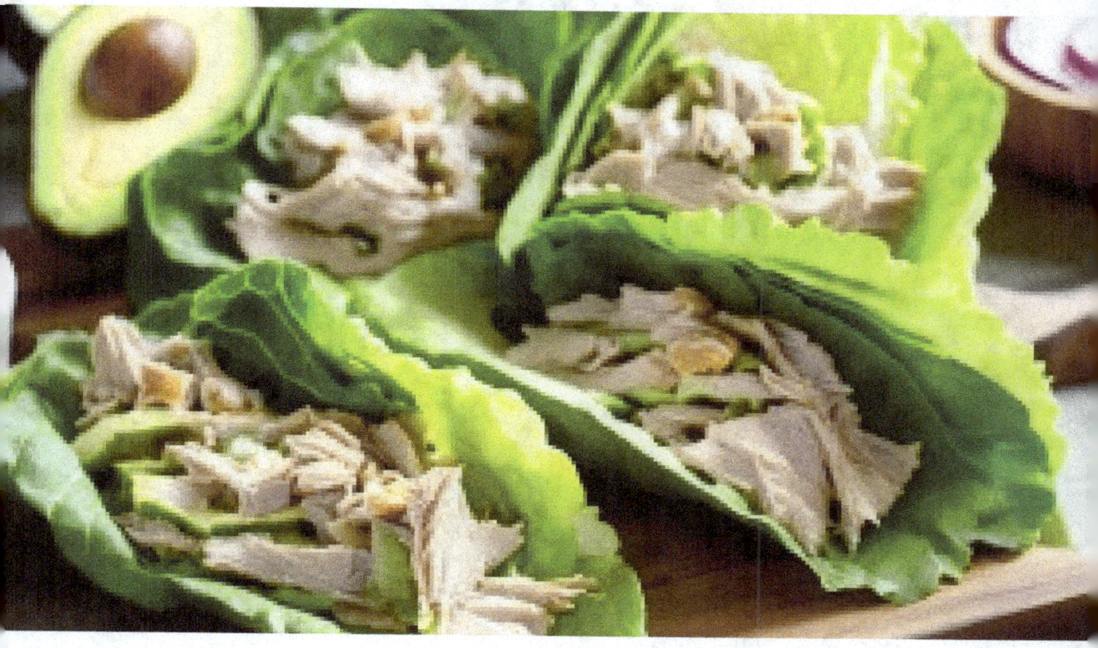

 2 Servings  5 minutes

INGREDIENTS

8 large lettuce leaves (such
as iceberg or butter lettuce)
8 slices deli turkey (Low-
FODMAP)
1 avocado, sliced
1/2 cup shredded carrots
Salt and pepper to taste

DIRECTIONS

1. Lay out lettuce leaves and top
   each with a slice of turkey,
   avocado slices, and shredded
   carrots.
2. Season with salt and pepper.
   Roll up and enjoy!

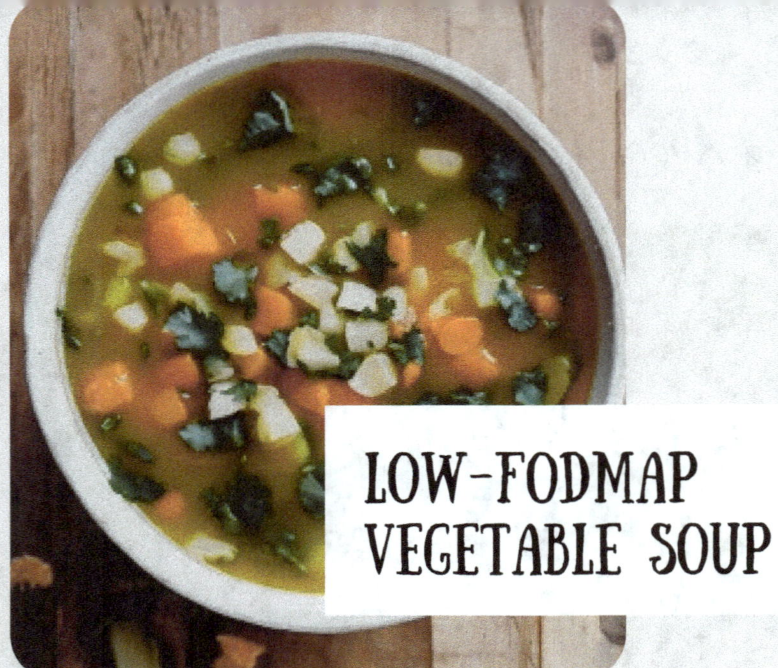

LOW-FODMAP VEGETABLE SOUP

SERVINGS: 4   TIME: 30 MINUTES

INGREDIENTS

1 tablespoon olive oil

2 carrots, diced

1 zucchini, diced

1/2 cup chopped green beans

4 cups vegetable broth

1 teaspoon dried thyme

Salt and pepper to taste

DIRECTIONS

1. Heat olive oil in a pot over medium heat. Add carrots, zucchini, and green beans. Cook for 5 minutes.
2. Add vegetable broth and thyme. Bring to a boil, then simmer for 20 minutes.
3. Season with salt and pepper before serving.

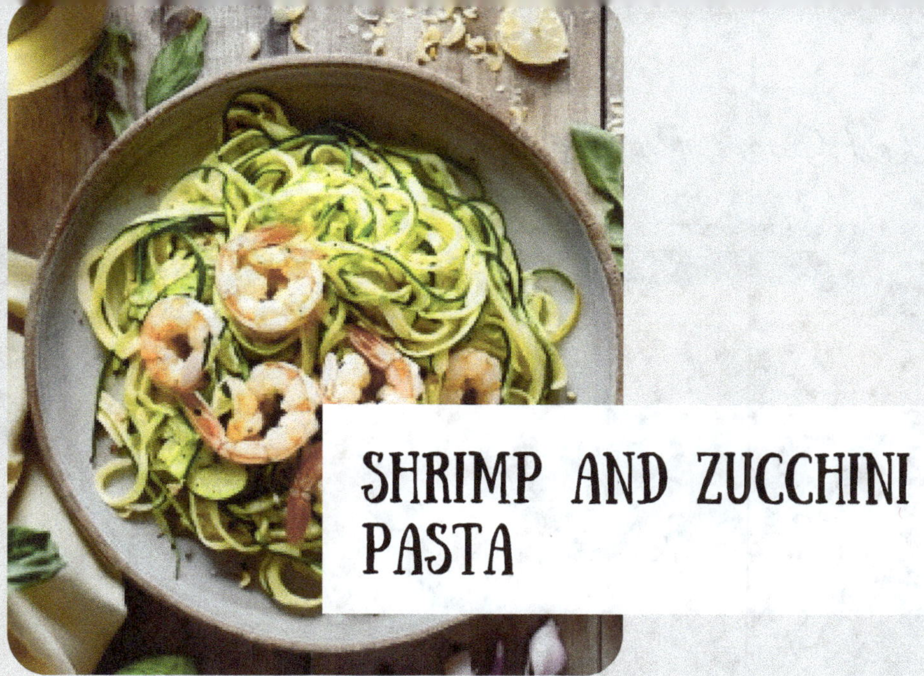

SHRIMP AND ZUCCHINI PASTA

SERVINGS: 2

TIME: 15 MINUTES

INGREDIENTS

8 ounces gluten-free
spaghetti
1 pound shrimp,
peeled and deveined
2 zucchinis, spiralized
into noodles
2 tablespoons olive oil
1 teaspoon dried
oregano
Salt and pepper to
taste

DIRECTIONS

1. Cook gluten-free spaghetti according to package instructions.
2. Heat olive oil in a pan over medium heat. Add shrimp, cooking until pink, about 3-4 minutes.
3. Add spiralized zucchini, cooked spaghetti, oregano, salt, and pepper. Toss to combine.

Baked Sweet Potato with Tuna

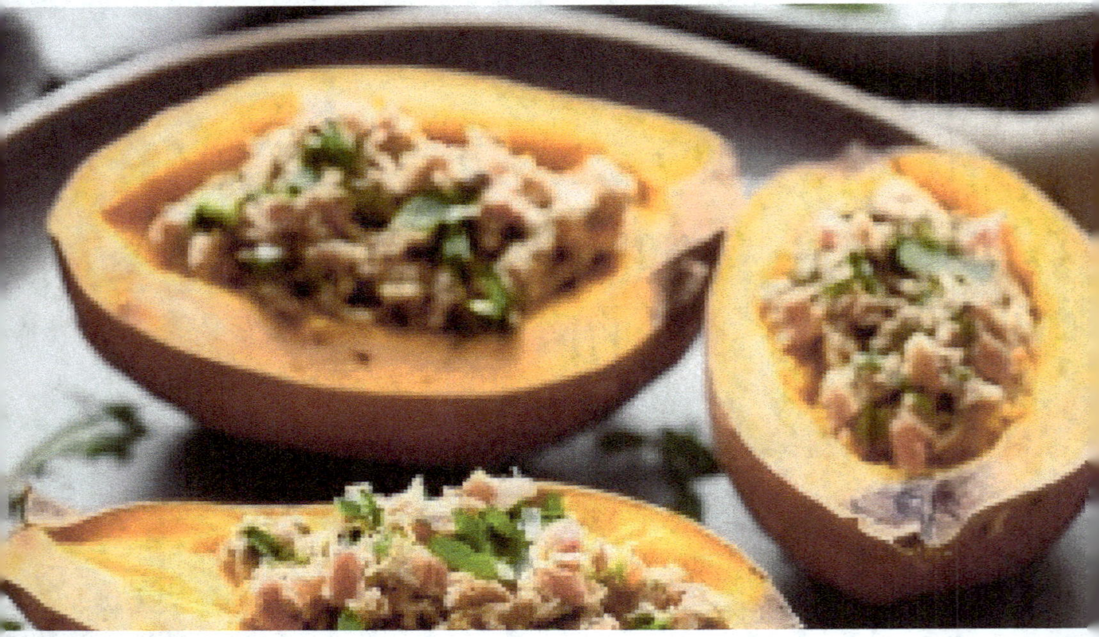

 2 Servings 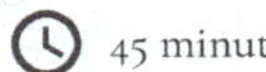 45 minutes

INGREDIENTS

2 medium sweet
potatoes
1 can tuna in olive oil,
drained
1/4 cup chopped green
onions (green parts
only)
Salt and pepper to taste

DIRECTIONS

1. Preheat oven to 400°F (200°C).
   Bake sweet potatoes for 40-45
   minutes, or until tender.
2. Split open the sweet potatoes
   and top with tuna and chopped
   green onions. Season with salt
   and pepper.

Greek Quinoa Salad

 4 servings   20 minutes

INGREDIENTS

1 cup cooked quinoa

1/2 cup diced cucumber

1/2 cup diced tomatoes

1/4 cup crumbled feta
(optional)

1/4 cup pitted black
olives, sliced

2 tablespoons olive oil

Juice of 1 lemon

Salt and pepper to taste

DIRECTIONS

1. In a large bowl, combine quinoa, cucumber, tomatoes, feta, and olives.
2. Drizzle with olive oil and lemon juice. Season with salt and pepper, and toss to combine.

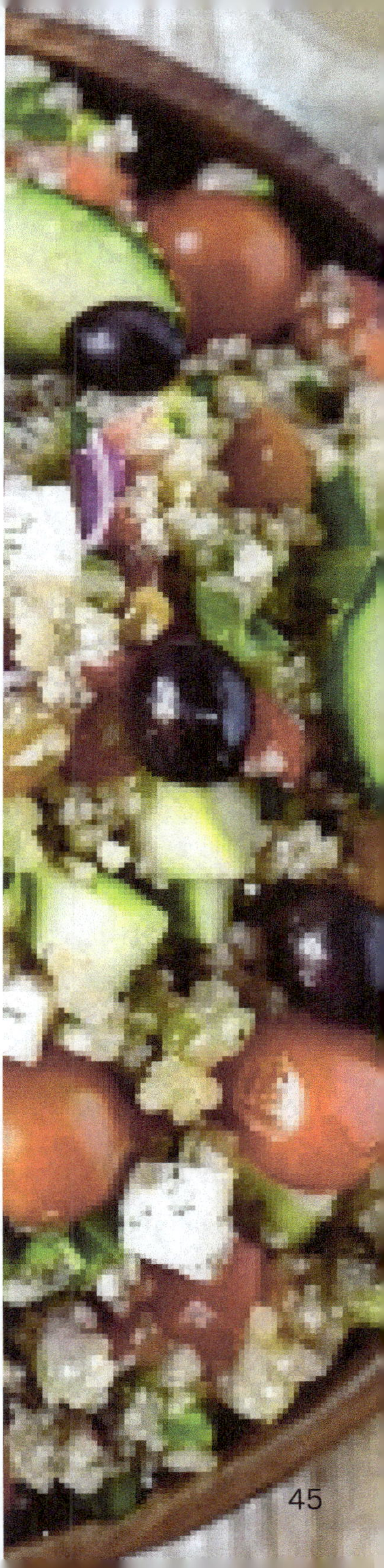

Egg Fried Rice

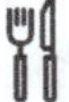 2 servings    10 minutes

INGREDIENTS

2 cups cooked and cooled
rice
2 large eggs, beaten
1/2 cup diced carrots
1/4 cup chopped scallions
(green parts only)
2 tablespoons tamari (gluten–
free soy sauce)
1 tablespoon sesame oil

DIRECTIONS

1. Heat sesame oil in a pan over
   medium heat. Add carrots and
   cook for 2–3 minutes.
2. Push carrots to one side and pour
   in beaten eggs, scrambling them.
3. Add cooked rice and tamari. Stir
   to combine and heat through.
   Garnish with scallions.

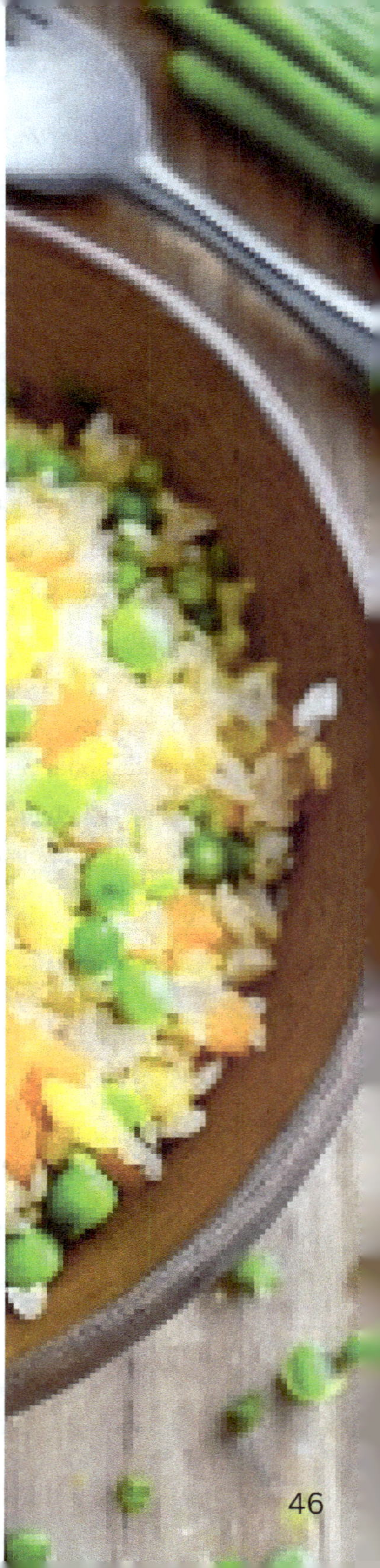

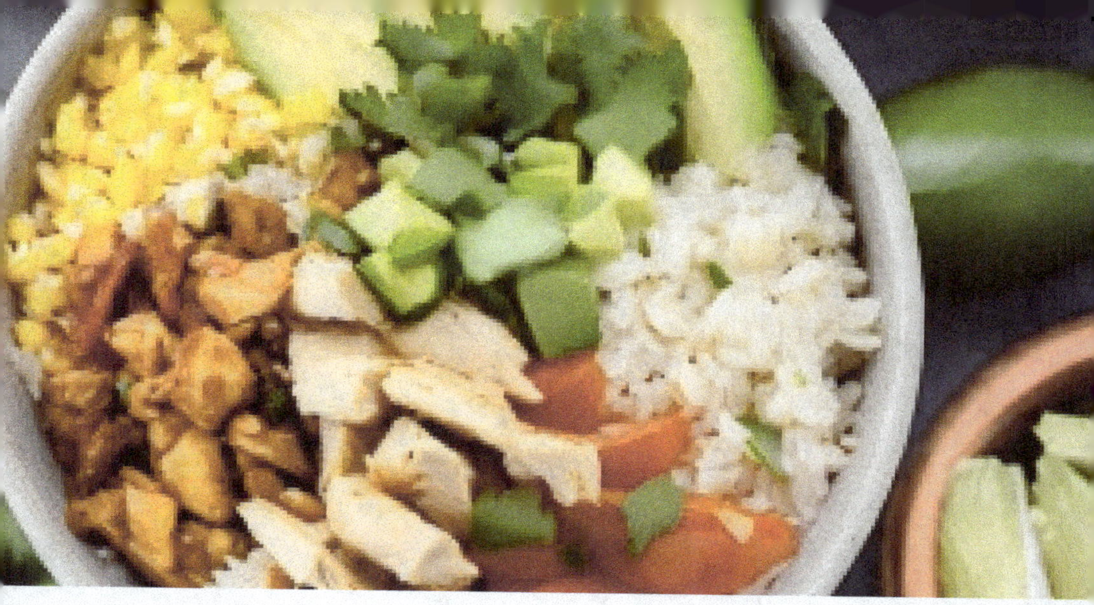

Chicken and Rice Burrito Bowl

Ingredients :

2 boneless, skinless chicken
breasts, cooked and sliced
2 cups cooked rice
1/2 cup diced bell peppers
1/2 cup shredded lettuce
1/4 cup lactose-free sour cream
1/4 cup shredded cheddar
cheese (optional)

Procedure :

1. Divide cooked rice between
two bowls.

2. Top with sliced chicken, bell
peppers, lettuce, sour cream,
and shredded cheese.

3. Serve immediately.

Prep Time : 20 minutes

Servings : 2

Chapter 6

DINNER RECIPES

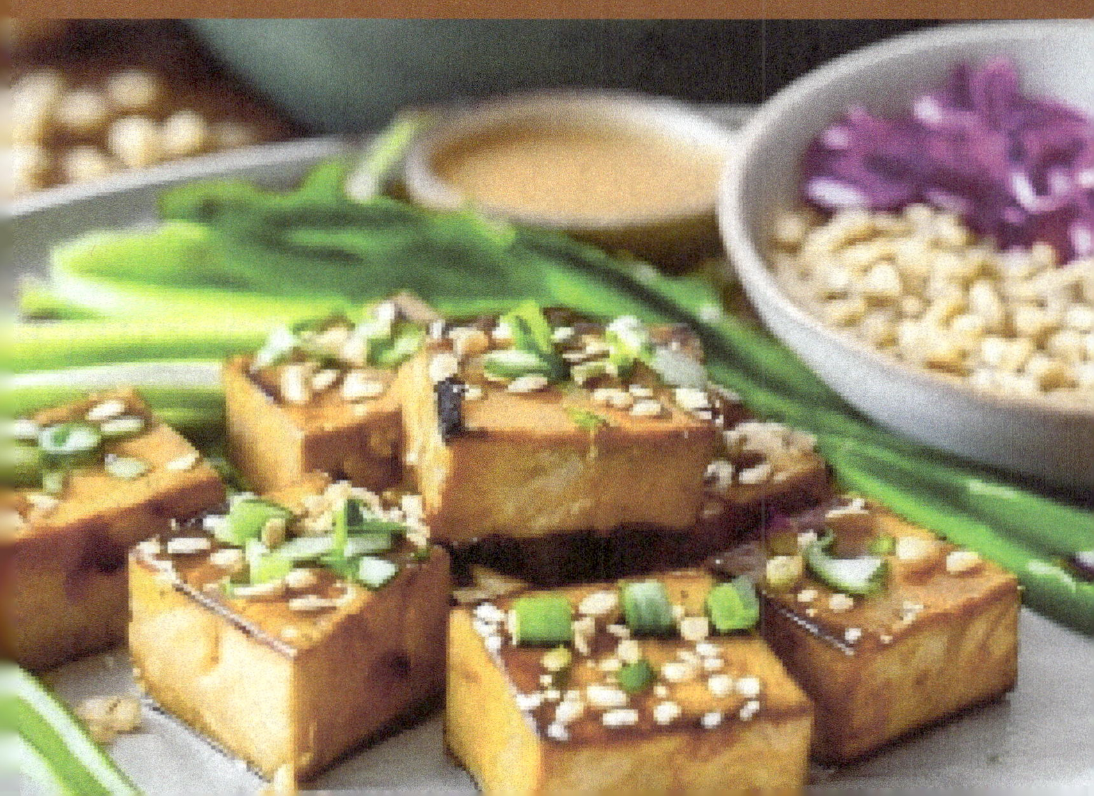

Lemon Garlic Shrimp Pasta

4 Servings   20 minutes

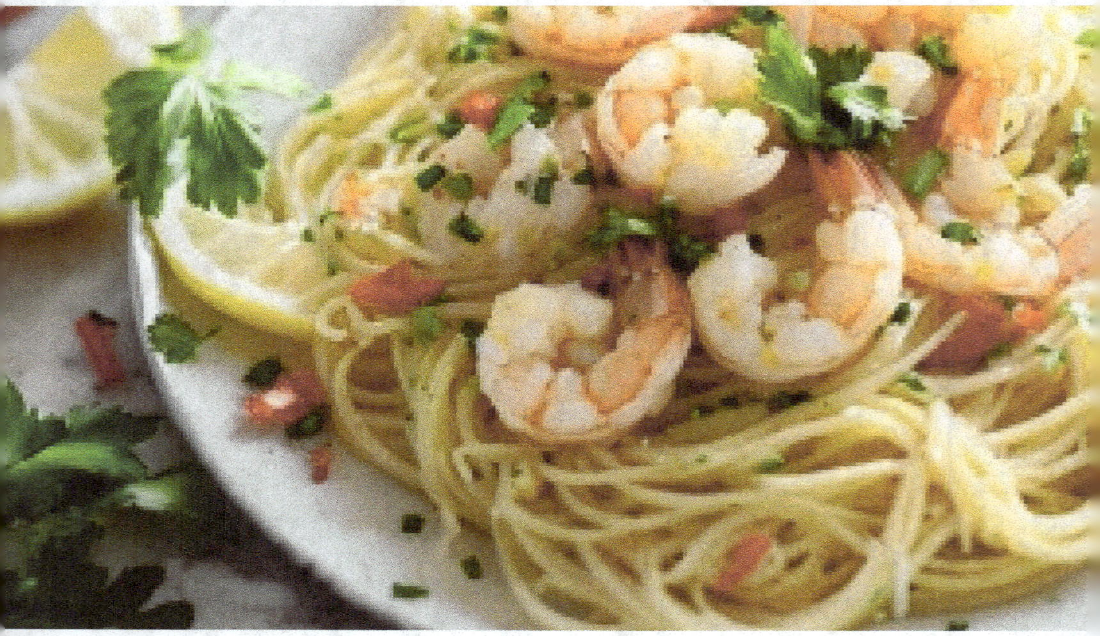

INGREDIENTS

8 ounces gluten-free spaghetti
1 pound shrimp, peeled and deveined
2 tablespoons olive oil
3 tablespoons lemon juice
2 tablespoons chopped fresh parsley
Salt and pepper to taste

DIRECTIONS

1. Cook gluten-free spaghetti according to package instructions.
2. Heat olive oil in a pan over medium heat. Add shrimp and cook until pink, about 3-4 minutes.
3. Add cooked pasta, lemon juice, parsley, salt, and pepper. Toss to combine and serve hot.

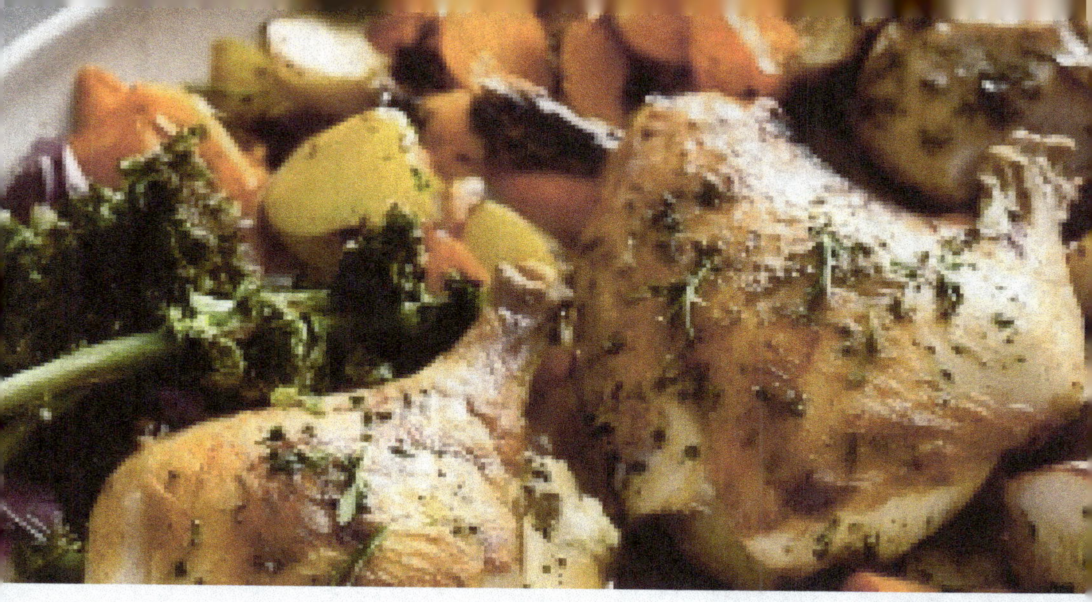

Herb-Roasted Chicken with Vegetables

Ingredients :

4 bone-in, skin-on chicken thighs
2 cups diced carrots
2 cups diced potatoes
1 tablespoon olive oil
1 teaspoon dried rosemary
1 teaspoon dried thyme
Salt and pepper to taste

Prep Time : 50 minutes

Servings : 4

Procedure :

1. Preheat the oven to 400°F (200°C).

2. Place chicken thighs, carrots, and potatoes on a baking sheet. Drizzle with olive oil and season with rosemary, thyme, salt, and pepper.

3. Roast for 45-50 minutes, or until the chicken is cooked through and vegetables are tender.

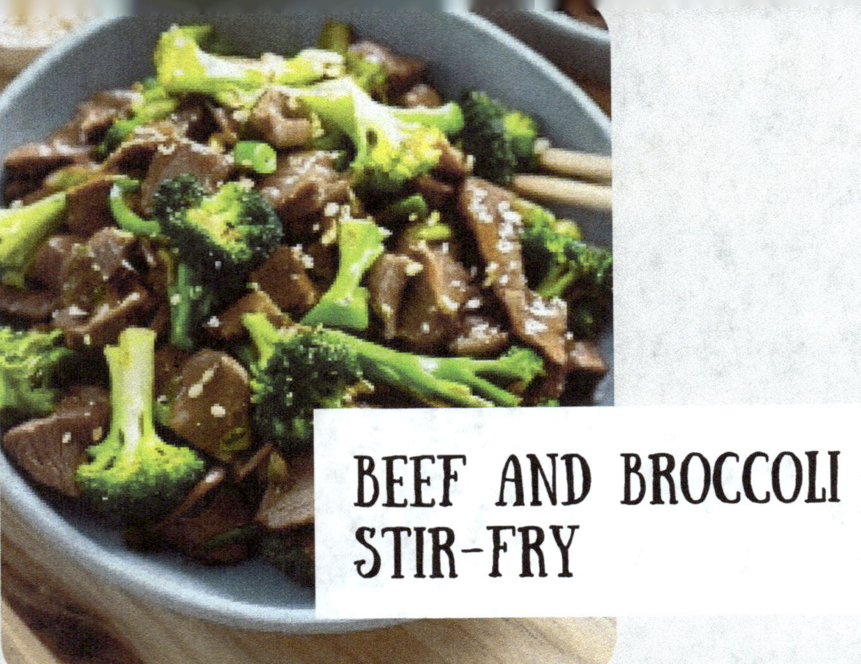

BEEF AND BROCCOLI STIR-FRY

SERVINGS: 4

TIME: 20 MINUTES

INGREDIENTS

1 pound flank steak, thinly sliced

2 cups broccoli florets

2 tablespoons tamari (gluten-free soy sauce)

1 tablespoon sesame oil

1 tablespoon cornstarch

Salt and pepper to taste

DIRECTIONS

1. Toss sliced beef with cornstarch, salt, and pepper.
2. Heat sesame oil in a pan over medium-high heat. Add beef and cook until browned, about 4-5 minutes.
3. Add broccoli and tamari, cooking until broccoli is tender. Serve immediately.

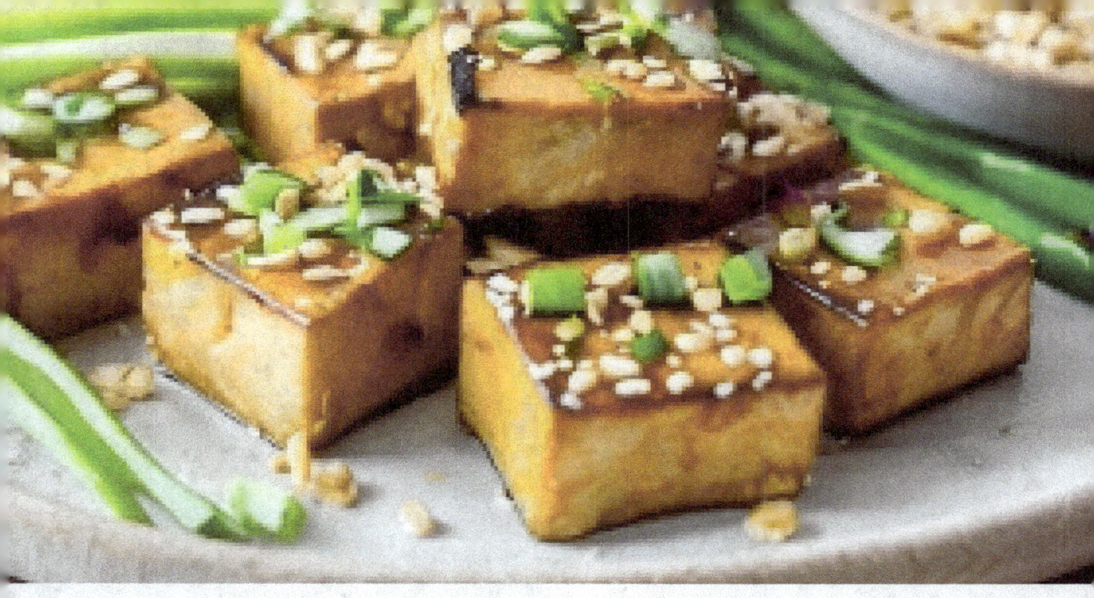

Crispy Baked Tofu with Peanut Sauce

Ingredients :

1 block firm tofu, cubed
2 tablespoons olive oil
1/4 cup peanut butter
2 tablespoons tamari (gluten-free soy sauce)
1 tablespoon lime juice
1 tablespoon honey (or maple syrup)

Procedure :

1. Preheat oven to 400°F (200°C). Toss tofu cubes with olive oil and spread on a baking sheet. Bake for 25 minutes, or until crispy.

2. In a bowl, mix peanut butter, tamari, lime juice, and honey. Drizzle over the baked tofu and serve.

Prep Time : 30 minutes

Servings : 4

Baked Salmon with Lemon and Dill

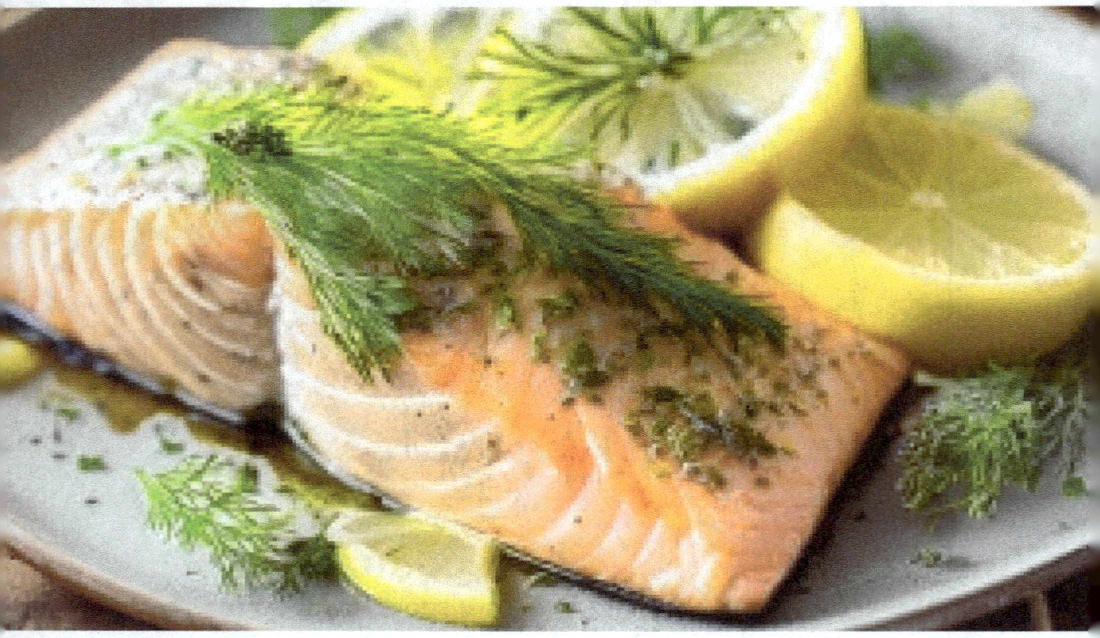

 2 Servings  15 minutes

INGREDIENTS

2 salmon fillets

1 tablespoon olive oil

Juice of 1 lemon

1 tablespoon chopped fresh dill

Salt and pepper to taste

DIRECTIONS

1. Preheat oven to 375°F (190°C).
2. Place salmon fillets on a baking sheet. Drizzle with olive oil and lemon juice, and sprinkle with dill, salt, and pepper.
3. Bake for 12–15 minutes, or until the salmon flakes easily with a fork.

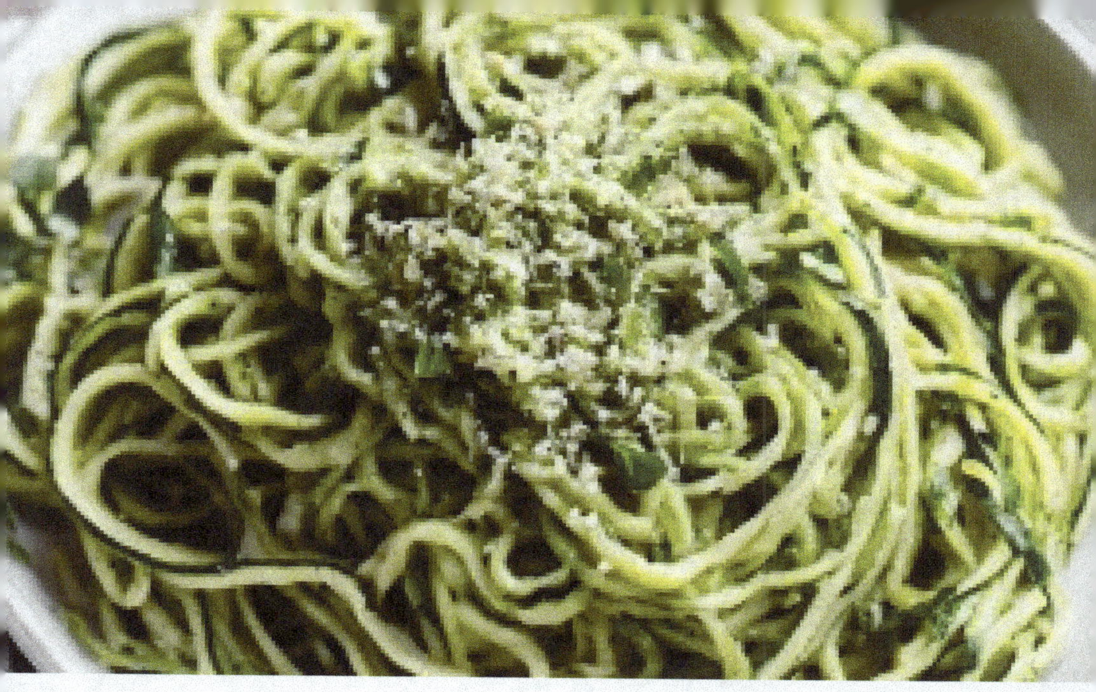

Zucchini Noodles with Pesto

Ingredients :

4 zucchinis, spiralized
1/2 cup lactose-free pesto
1/4 cup grated Parmesan
cheese
Salt and pepper to taste

Procedure :

1. Heat a large skillet over medium heat. Add spiralized zucchini and cook for 3-4 minutes.

2. Stir in pesto and Parmesan cheese. Season with salt and pepper.

Prep Time : 15 minutes

Servings : 4

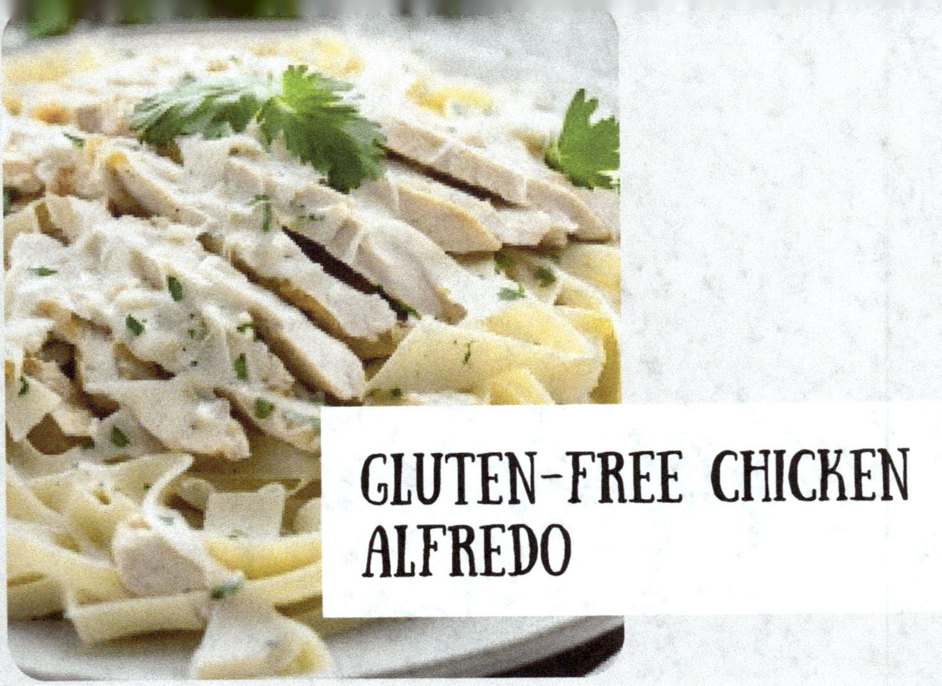

GLUTEN-FREE CHICKEN ALFREDO

SERVINGS: 4

TIME: 25 MINUTES

INGREDIENTS

2 boneless, skinless chicken breasts, sliced

8 ounces gluten-free fettuccine

1 cup lactose-free heavy cream

1/2 cup grated Parmesan cheese

2 tablespoons olive oil

Salt and pepper to taste

DIRECTIONS

1. Cook gluten-free fettuccine according to package instructions.
2. Heat olive oil in a skillet over medium heat. Add sliced chicken and cook until browned.
3. Stir in lactose-free heavy cream and Parmesan cheese, cooking until the sauce thickens. Toss with cooked pasta and serve.

Baked Cod with Fresh Herbs

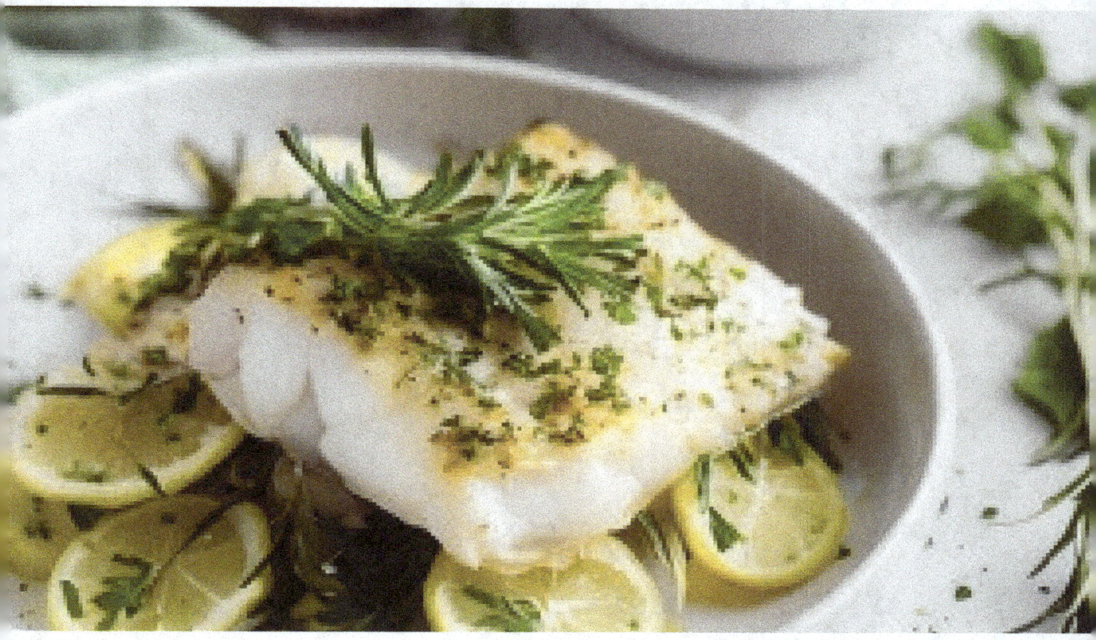

 4 Servings  20 minutes

INGREDIENTS

4 cod fillets
2 tablespoons olive oil
2 tablespoons chopped
fresh herbs (parsley,
dill, or chives)
Juice of 1 lemon
Salt and pepper to taste

DIRECTIONS

1. Preheat oven to 375°F (190°C).
2. Place cod fillets on a baking sheet. Drizzle with olive oil and lemon juice, and sprinkle with fresh herbs, salt, and pepper.
3. Bake for 15–20 minutes, or until the fish flakes easily with a fork.

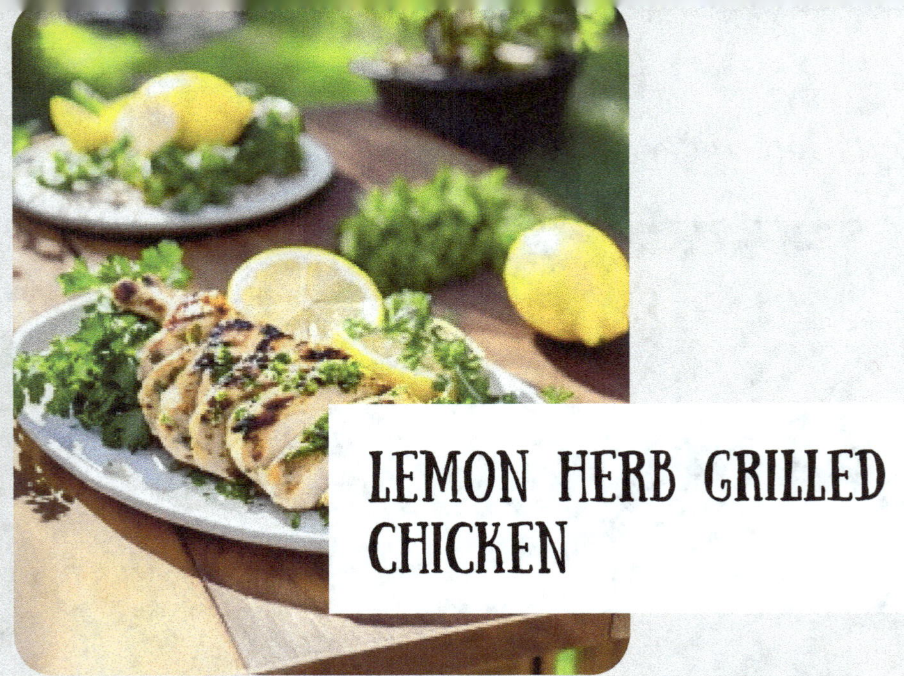

LEMON HERB GRILLED CHICKEN

SERVINGS: 4   TIME: 30 MINUTES (PLUS MARINATING TIME)

INGREDIENTS

4 boneless, skinless
chicken breasts
Juice of 2 lemons
2 tablespoons olive oil
2 tablespoons
chopped fresh herbs
(parsley, rosemary, or
thyme)
Salt and pepper to
taste

DIRECTIONS

1. Marinate chicken breasts in lemon juice, olive oil, herbs, salt, and pepper for at least 30 minutes.
2. Grill over medium heat for 6–7 minutes per side, or until fully cooked.

One-Pot Vegetable Curry

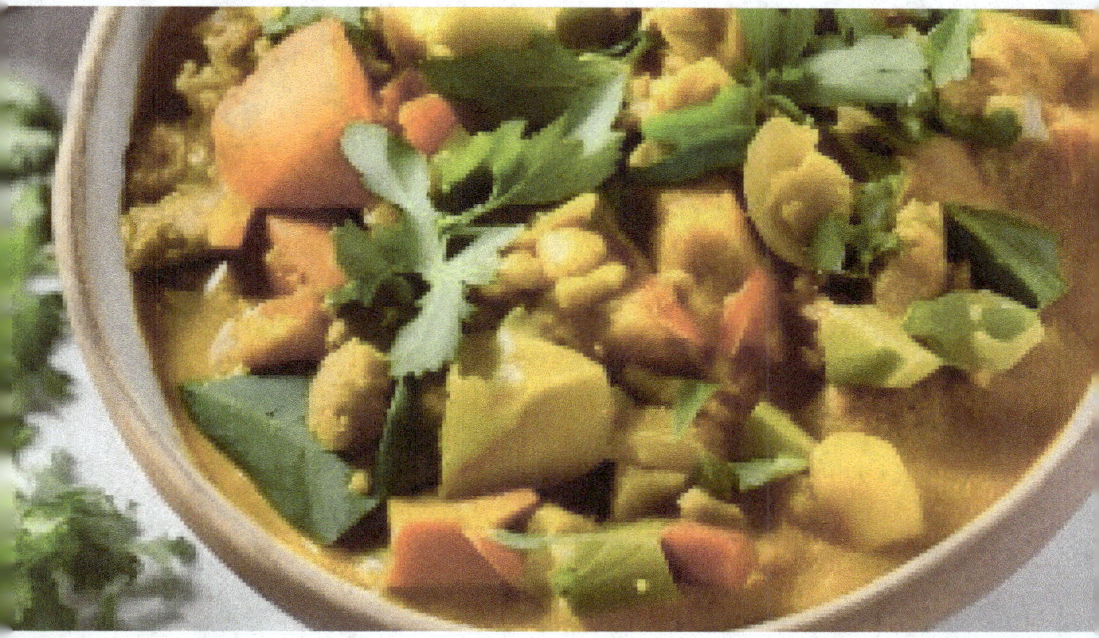

 4 Servings 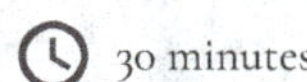 30 minutes

INGREDIENTS

2 tablespoons olive oil

1 cup diced potatoes

1 cup diced carrots

1 zucchini, sliced

1 can coconut milk

2 tablespoons curry powder

Salt and pepper to taste

DIRECTIONS

1. Heat olive oil in a large pot. Add potatoes, carrots, and zucchini, cooking until tender.
2. Stir in coconut milk and curry powder. Simmer for 15-20 minutes, or until vegetables are fully cooked. Season with salt and pepper.

Stuffed Bell Peppers

 4 servings   🕐 40 minutes

INGREDIENTS

4 large bell peppers,
halved and seeded
1 pound ground turkey
1 cup cooked rice
1 can diced tomatoes
(drained)
1 teaspoon dried
oregano
Salt and pepper to taste

DIRECTIONS

1. Preheat oven to 375°F (190°C).
2. In a skillet, cook ground turkey over medium heat until browned. Add cooked rice, diced tomatoes, oregano, salt, and pepper.
3. Stuff each bell pepper half with the turkey mixture. Place in a baking dish and bake for 30-35 minutes.

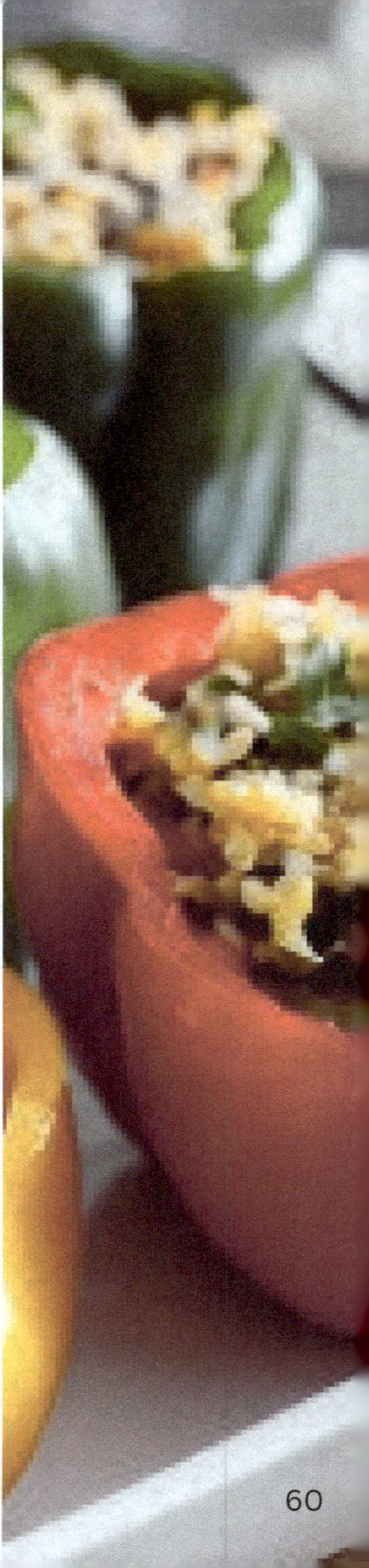

Chapter 7

Snacks and Treats

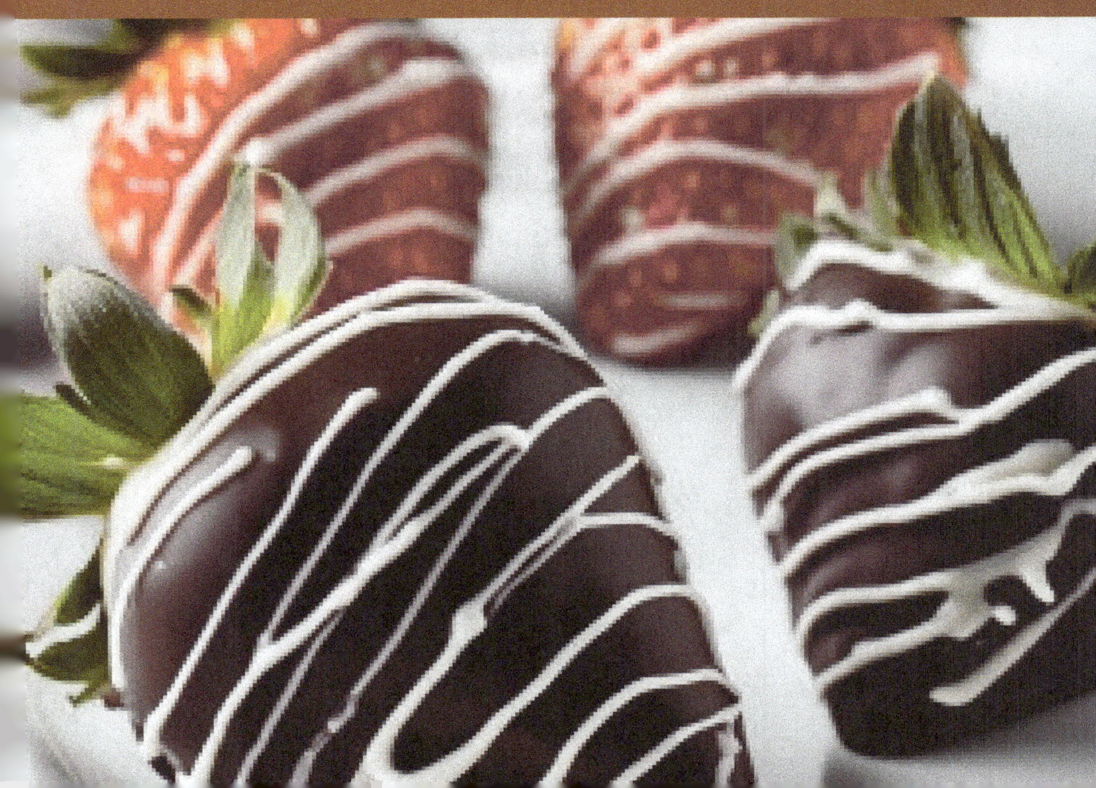

Low-FODMAP Hummus with Carrot Sticks

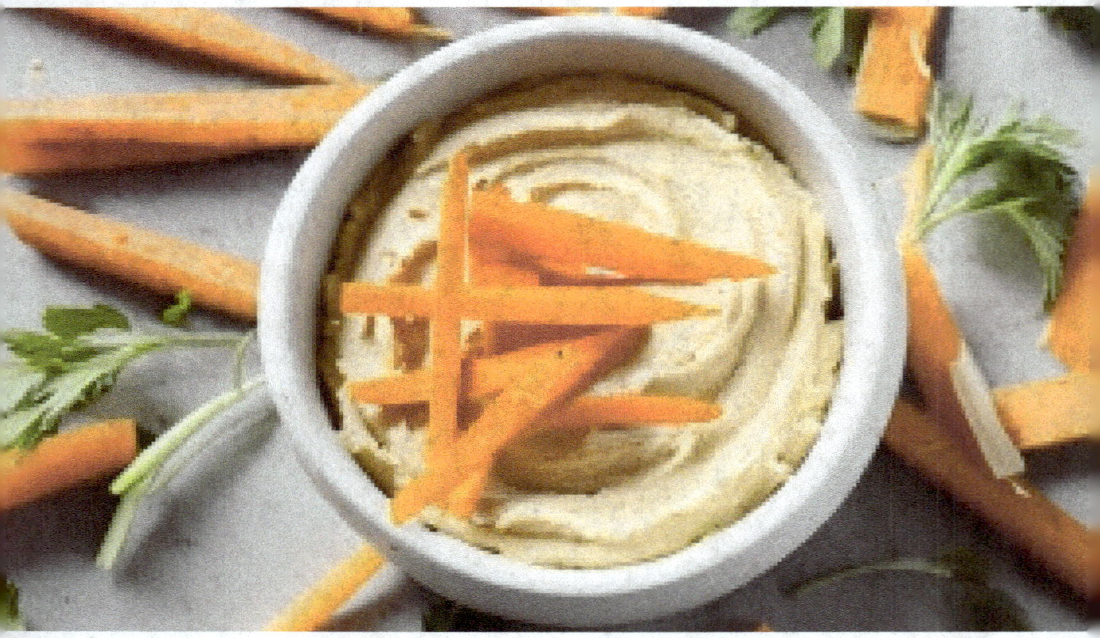

 4 Servings   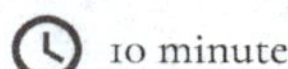 10 minutes

INGREDIENTS

1 can chickpeas,
drained and rinsed
2 tablespoons tahini
1/4 cup olive oil
Juice of 1 lemon
Salt and pepper to
taste
4 large carrots, cut
into sticks

DIRECTIONS

1. In a blender or food processor,
   blend chickpeas, tahini, olive oil,
   lemon juice, salt, and pepper
   until smooth.
2. Serve with carrot sticks.

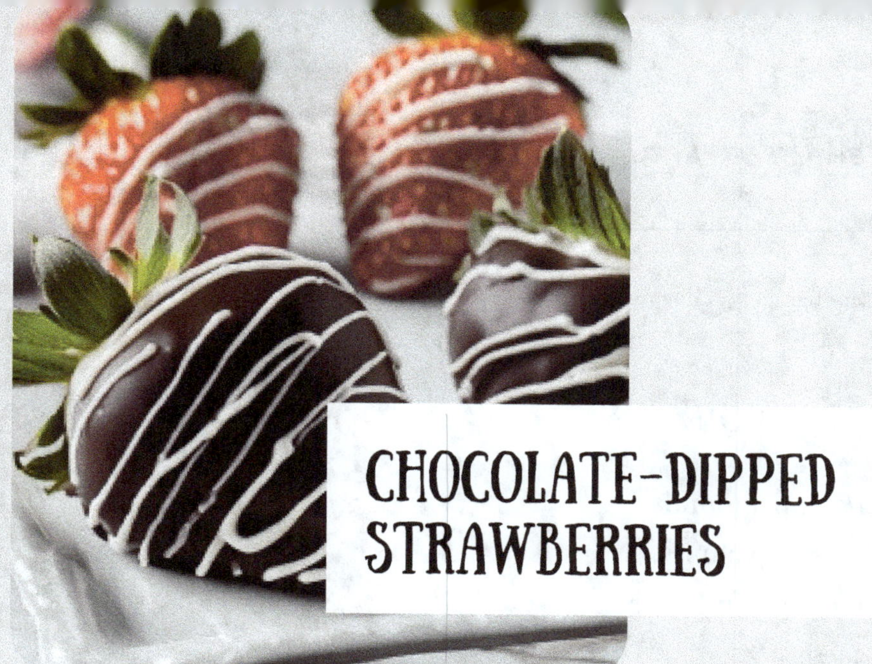

CHOCOLATE-DIPPED STRAWBERRIES

SERVINGS: 10 STRAWBERRIES

TIME: 10 MINUTES (PLUS CHILLING TIME)

INGREDIENTS

10 large strawberries

1/2 cup dark chocolate chips

DIRECTIONS

1. Melt dark chocolate chips in a microwave-safe bowl, stirring every 30 seconds until smooth.
2. Dip each strawberry into the melted chocolate and place on a lined baking sheet.
3. Refrigerate until the chocolate hardens, about 15 minutes.

Gluten-Free Trail Mix

 4 servings   5 minutes

INGREDIENTS

1/2 cup almonds

1/2 cup walnuts

1/4 cup sunflower
seeds

1/4 cup dried
cranberries (Low-
FODMAP portion)

1/4 cup dark
chocolate chips

DIRECTIONS

1. Combine all ingredients in a large
bowl.
2. Divide into small snack-sized
portions for an easy grab-and-go
treat.

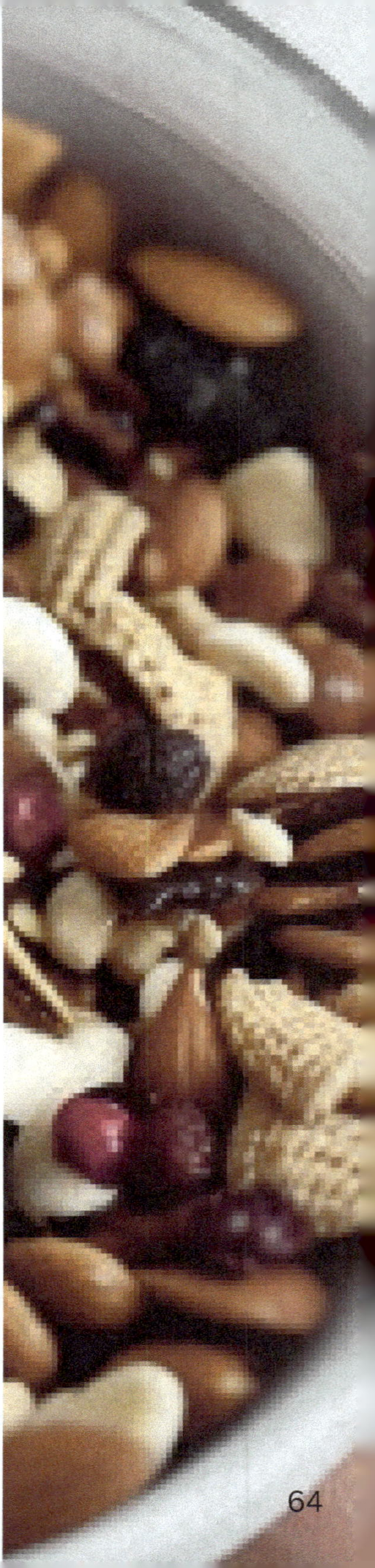

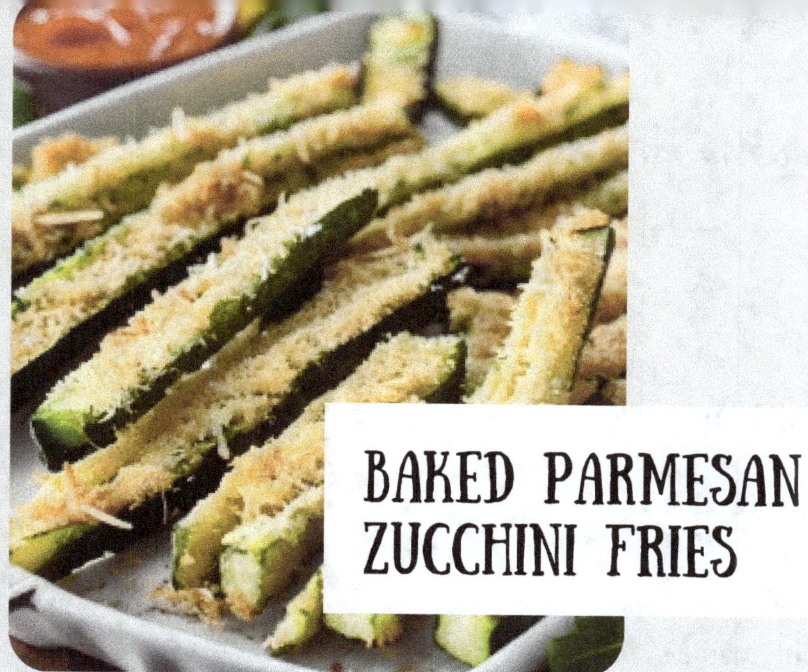

BAKED PARMESAN ZUCCHINI FRIES

SERVINGS: 4

TIME: 25 MINUTES

INGREDIENTS

2 large zucchinis, cut
into fries
1/2 cup grated
Parmesan cheese
1 tablespoon olive oil
Salt and pepper to
taste

DIRECTIONS

1. Preheat oven to 400°F (200°C) and line a baking sheet with parchment paper.
2. Toss zucchini fries with olive oil, Parmesan cheese, salt, and pepper.
3. Arrange on the baking sheet and bake for 20–25 minutes, or until golden and crispy.

Coconut Macaroons

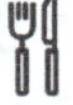 12 macaroons   🕐 20 minutes

INGREDIENTS

2 cups shredded
coconut
2 large egg whites
1/4 cup maple syrup
1 teaspoon vanilla
extract

DIRECTIONS

1. Preheat oven to 350°F (175°C) and line a baking sheet with parchment paper.
2. In a bowl, mix shredded coconut, egg whites, maple syrup, and vanilla extract until combined.
3. Scoop small mounds onto the baking sheet and bake for 15–20 minutes, or until golden brown.

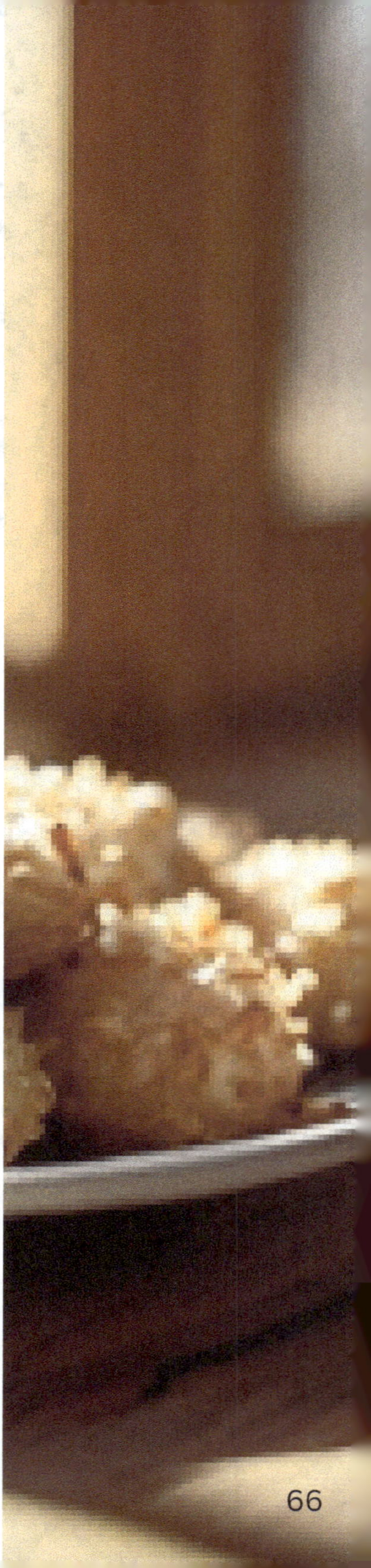

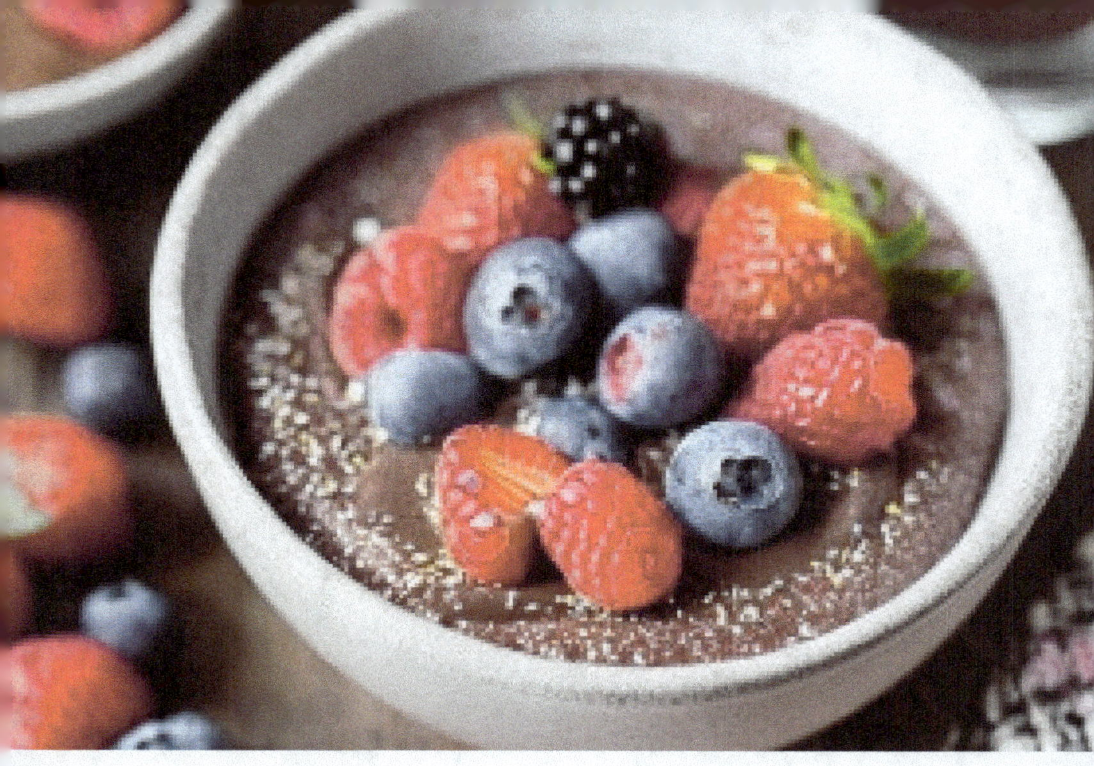

Low-FODMAP Chocolate Chia Pudding

Ingredients :

1/4 cup chia seeds

1 1/2 cups lactose-free milk
or almond milk

2 tablespoons cocoa powder

2 tablespoons maple syrup

Procedure :

1. In a bowl, mix chia seeds, lactose-free milk, cocoa powder, and maple syrup.

2. Stir well and refrigerate overnight. Serve chilled.

Prep Time : 5 minutes
(plus overnight chilling)

Servings : 2

Zucchini Chips

 4 Servings  2 hours

INGREDIENTS

2 large zucchinis,
thinly sliced
2 tablespoons olive oil
Salt and pepper to
taste

DIRECTIONS

1. Preheat oven to 225°F (110°C) and line a baking sheet with parchment paper.
2. Toss zucchini slices with olive oil, salt, and pepper.
3. Arrange in a single layer on the baking sheet and bake for 2 hours, or until crisp.

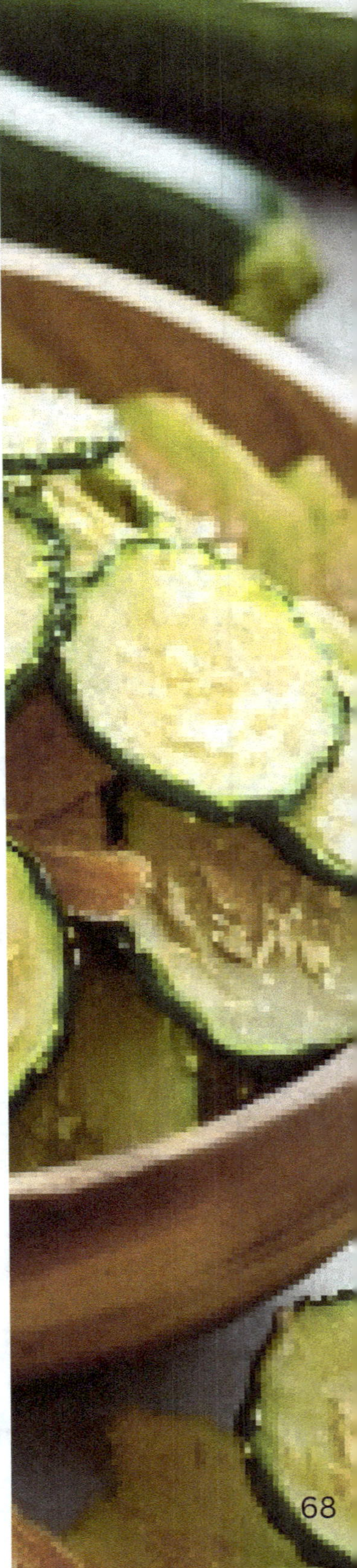

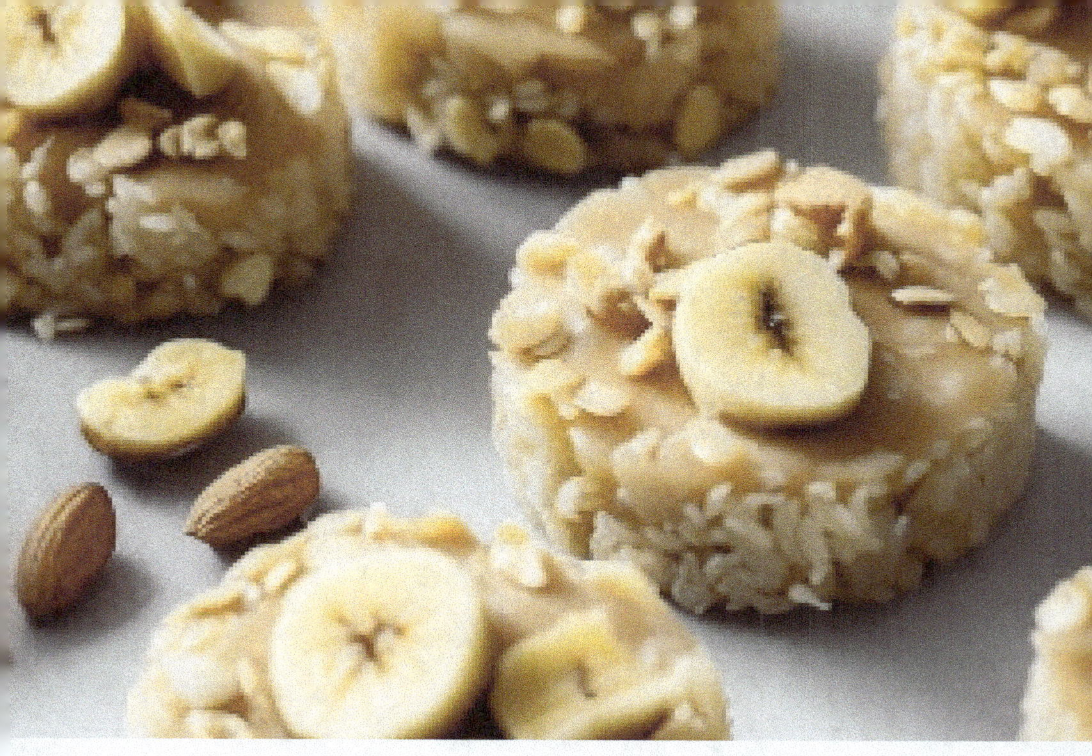

Banana and Peanut Butter Rice Cakes

Ingredients :

2 rice cakes

1 ripe banana, sliced

2 tablespoons peanut butter

A sprinkle of cinnamon

Procedure :

1. Spread peanut butter over each rice cake.

2. Top with banana slices and a sprinkle of cinnamon. Serve immediately.

Prep Time : 5 minutes

Servings : 2

CHAPTER 8

EATING OUT AND TRAVELING MADE EASY

Following a Low-FODMAP Diet doesn't mean you have to miss out on the joy of dining out or the thrill of traveling. While it may seem daunting at first, with a little bit of planning and the right strategies, you can still enjoy meals away from home without compromising your gut health. Let's explore how you can confidently navigate social situations and travel while staying on track with your diet.

Choosing Low-FODMAP Options at Restaurants

Eating out at restaurants can feel intimidating when you're trying to avoid FODMAPs, but you can still enjoy delicious meals with the right approach. Here are some tips to make your dining experience stress-free:

1. **Research Before You Go:** Before heading to a restaurant, take a look at their menu online. Many restaurants have detailed menus and even list allergen information. If you can't find what you need, don't hesitate to call ahead and ask about Low-FODMAP options.

2. **Pick Simple Dishes:** Choose meals that are made with whole, unprocessed ingredients. Grilled meats, fish, or tofu served with plain rice, baked potatoes, or simple steamed vegetables are generally safe choices.

3. **Customize Your Order:** Don't be afraid to ask for modifications to your meal. Request that your dish be prepared without high-FODMAP ingredients like garlic, onions, or rich sauces. For salads, ask for dressing on the side and choose a simple oil and vinegar option.

4. **Bring Your Own Condiments:** If you're unsure about the ingredients in sauces or dressings, consider bringing your own. Small packets of olive oil, vinegar, or Low-FODMAP salad dressing can be lifesavers when dining out.

5. **Communicate Clearly with Your Server:** Explain your dietary needs politely but clearly. Instead of using medical terms or the word "FODMAP," which may be unfamiliar, simply state that you have food sensitivities and specify the ingredients you need to avoid. Most restaurants are happy to accommodate your requests.

6. **Choose International Cuisines Wisely:** Some types of cuisine are more Low-FODMAP-friendly than others. For example, Japanese cuisine often features simple grilled meats and sushi made with rice and fresh fish. Mexican cuisine can be a good option if you stick to corn tortillas, grilled meats, and simple salsas (without onions or garlic).

STAYING ON TRACK WHILE AWAY FROM HOME

Traveling can be one of the most challenging aspects of following a Low-FODMAP Diet, but with some smart planning, you can stay on track and enjoy your trip. Here's how to make your travels enjoyable and worry-free:

1. **Pack Low-FODMAP Snacks:** When you're on the go, having snacks readily available can save you from making poor food choices. Some great travel-friendly options include rice cakes, peanut butter packets, gluten-free granola bars, Low-FODMAP trail mix, and fresh fruit like bananas or oranges.

2. **Book Accommodations with a Kitchen:** If possible, choose accommodations that allow you to prepare your own meals.

Having access to a small kitchen or kitchenette gives you more control over what you eat and makes it easy to prepare simple, Low-FODMAP meals.

3. **Research Local Grocery Stores:** Before you arrive at your destination, research nearby grocery stores or markets where you can buy fresh, Low-FODMAP ingredients. Stocking up on essentials like lactose-free milk, gluten-free bread, and safe proteins will make your stay much easier.

4. **Plan Ahead for Flights and Road Trips:** Airport and rest stop food can be limited, so pack a meal or snacks to take with you. If you're flying, be sure to check the airline's meal options in advance or bring your own meal to avoid any surprises.

5. **Download Helpful Apps:** Use apps that can help you identify Low-FODMAP-friendly restaurants and meals. Apps like FODMAP-specific food guides or restaurant finders can make eating out while traveling much more manageable.

6. **Stay Hydrated:** Traveling often means spending long hours on planes or in cars, which can lead to dehydration. Drink plenty of water and avoid sugary or carbonated beverages, as they can exacerbate digestive issues.

7. **Be Flexible and Prepared for the Unexpected:** Despite your best efforts, there may be times when you can't find perfectly Low-FODMAP options. If this happens, try to make the best choice available and don't stress too much about a minor slip-up. Your body is resilient, and one meal won't undo your overall progress.

Sample Low-FODMAP Travel-Friendly Snacks

To help you plan ahead, here are some snack ideas that are easy to pack and travel well:

- **Rice Cakes with Peanut Butter:** A simple and satisfying snack that requires no refrigeration.
- **Lactose-Free Cheese and Gluten-Free Crackers:** A portable and filling option for long days.
- **Low-FODMAP Trail Mix:** Combine almonds, walnuts, sunflower seeds, and a handful of dried cranberries for a healthy snack.
- **Fresh Fruit:** Bananas, oranges, or blueberries are easy to pack and provide a quick energy boost.
- **Instant Oatmeal Packets:** Choose plain, gluten-free oatmeal packets that you can mix with hot water for a quick breakfast or snack.

Final Thoughts

Eating out and traveling don't have to derail your Low-FODMAP Diet. With thoughtful planning and a proactive mindset, you can enjoy delicious meals and new experiences while keeping your gut happy. Remember, the goal is to enjoy life and feel your best—so don't be afraid to take control, make special requests, and pack your favorite snacks.

Enjoy your meals and your adventures, knowing that you have the tools to stay on track!

ACKNOWLEDGMENTS

Writing this book has been a journey filled with growth, learning, and deep appreciation for the people who made it possible. First and foremost, I would like to express my sincere gratitude to my readers. Your dedication to improving your health and well-being inspires me every day, and I hope this book provides you with the support and guidance you need to thrive.

To my family and friends, thank you for your support and encouragement. Your patience, love, and belief in me kept me motivated and focused throughout this project. A special thanks to [mention specific family members or friends if desired] for your understanding and for always cheering me on.

I would also like to acknowledge the invaluable contributions of my healthcare and nutrition experts. To [mention specific dietitians, doctors, or other professionals], thank you for sharing your expertise and helping to shape the information in this book. Your insights and guidance have made this work not only accurate but also accessible and practical for those navigating the challenges of digestive health.

A heartfelt thank you goes to my editor and publishing team. Your dedication to bringing this book to life with clarity and precision has been instrumental. To [mention specific individuals from the publishing team], your hard work, attention to detail, and commitment to excellence have not gone unnoticed.

Lastly, to all the researchers and pioneers in the field of Low-FODMAP nutrition, thank you for your tireless efforts to advance our understanding of gut health. Your groundbreaking work has provided a foundation for this book and for the many people who have found relief and hope through the Low-FODMAP Diet.

This book is a testament to the power of collaboration and shared knowledge. Thank you to everyone, I am deeply grateful.

www.ingramcontent.com/pod-product-compliance
Lightning Source LLC
Chambersburg PA
CBHW061516250726
48657CB00005B/1903